THE INTELLIGENT CLINICIAN'S GUIDE TO DSM-5®

THE INTELLIGENT
CLINICIAN'S GUIDE TO DSM-5®

Joel Paris, MD

PROFESSOR OF PSYCHIATRY

McGILL UNIVERSITY

MONTREAL, CANADA

OXFORD

UNIVERSITY PRESS

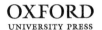

OXFORD
UNIVERSITY PRESS

Oxford University Press is a department of the University of Oxford.
It furthers the University's objective of excellence in research, scholarship,
and education by publishing worldwide.

Oxford   New York
Auckland   Cape Town   Dar es Salaam   Hong Kong   Karachi
Kuala Lumpur   Madrid   Melbourne   Mexico City   Nairobi
New Delhi   Shanghai   Taipei   Toronto

With offices in
Argentina   Austria   Brazil   Chile   Czech Republic   France   Greece
Guatemala   Hungary   Italy   Japan   Poland   Portugal   Singapore
South Korea   Switzerland   Thailand   Turkey   Ukraine   Vietnam

Oxford is a registered trademark of Oxford University Press
in the UK and certain other countries.

Published in the United States of America by
Oxford University Press
198 Madison Avenue, New York, NY 10016

Library of Congress Cataloging-in-Publication Data
Paris, Joel, 1940–
The intelligent clinician's guide to the DSM-5 / Joel Paris.
p. ; cm.
Includes bibliographical references and index.
ISBN 978–0–19–973817–5 (pbk. : alk. paper)
I. Title.
[DNLM: 1. Diagnostic and statistical manual of mental disorders. 5th ed.
2. Mental Disorders—diagnosis.   3. Mental Disorders—classification. WM 141]
616.89—dc23
2012040612

5 7 9 8 6 4
Printed in the United States of America
on acid-free paper

Disclosure statement: Joel Paris has no competing interests.

This book is dedicated to the memory of
Heinz Lehmann—teacher, research pioneer, and skeptic.

CONTENTS

PART THREE
OVERVIEW

INTRODUCTION

2013 marks the publication of DSM-5, the 5th edition of the Diagnostic and Statistical Manual of Mental Disorders (DSM), published by the American Psychiatric Association (APA). This is the first major revision in more than 30 years. In the past, the diagnosis of mental disorders was an abstruse subject, of interest only to researchers and a few experts. But mental disorders, as medical diagnoses, require scientific classification. Today, the DSM system has a profound influence on all the mental health professions. Revisions of psychiatry's diagnostic manual are front-page news.

DSM-5 will be a landmark for psychiatry, but understanding it requires time and attention to details. This book will be a guide to the main features of the new manual. It will focus on three questions. First, what are the most important changes? Second, what are the implications of these changes for practice? Third, is DSM-5 better, worse, or equal to its predecessors? This book, as a critical guide for the intelligent clinician, will applaud the positive aspects of DSM-5 but underline its limitations. It will be supportive of some changes but critical of others.

WHAT DSM-5 CAN AND CANNOT DO

The first two manuals published by APA, DSM-I (1952) and DSM-II (1968), did not have a great impact on psychiatry. In contrast, the third edition of the manual, DSM-III, published in 1980, was a major break with the past and a best-selling book. It moved classification from clinical impressions to a degree of rigor. It increased reliability by taking an "atheoretical" position—that is, making diagnoses based on what clinicians can see and agree on, rather than on abstract theories. DSM-III, and its successors, found a place on the shelf of almost every psychiatrist, psychologist, and mental health professional. There have been only minor changes over the last 30 years. The most recent revision (DSM-IV-TR) has been in place since 2000. Now changes in DSM-5 will require clinicians to relearn how to classify and conceptualize some mental disorders.

Is the DSM-5 system an improvement? One would like to believe so, and there are a number of places where it is. But there are problems. Some derive from the concept that psychopathology lies on a continuum with normality. This makes it difficult to separate mental disorders from normal variations, and therefore runs the danger of overdiagnosis. Other problems derive from the principle that mental disorders are brain disorders. Although great progress has been made over the last few decades, and although neuroscience has explained much about the brain, the origins of mental illness remain a mystery. No brain scan can explain why people develop schizophrenia, mania, or depression. Morever, although revisions in the manual are necessary, we do not yet know enough to develop a classification firmly based on data. If we don't know enough, then we should not invest in change for change's sake. Sometimes it is better to keep a known system, however faulty, than make modifications with unpredictable consequences. Even the smallest changes to diagnostic criteria can have profound effects on research and practice. Finally, some revisions lack clinical utility. Revising DSM is an enormous job, and each edition has grown larger, more complicated, and thicker. Much of what is written in the manual will never be applied in practice.

THE VALIDITY OF PSYCHIATRIC DIAGNOSIS

DSM-III made diagnosis more reliable, but reliability is not validity. Over the last 33 years, constant use of the DSM manuals has given clinicians the impression that the categories they describe must be valid. That is not true. DSM-5 lacks the data to define mental disorders in the way that physicians conceptualize medical illnesses. Some diagnoses in medicine are also vague, but psychiatry is far behind other specialties in grounding categories in measurements independent of clinical observation.

Almost all DSM diagnoses are based entirely on signs and symptoms. Some disorders have attracted more research, providing at least some support for validity, and although observation can be made more precise through statistical evaluation and expert consensus, other areas of medicine use blood tests, imaging, or genetic markers to confirm impressions drawn from signs and symptoms. Psychiatry is nowhere near that level of knowledge. No biological markers or tests exist for *any* diagnosis in psychiatry. For this reason, any claim that DSM-5 is more scientific than its predecessors is little but hype.

In 1980, I was a strong supporter of the paradigm shift introduced by DSM-III. It was progressive to move classification away from unproven theories and to make diagnosis dependent on observation. But this was a provisional stance that became frozen in time, and progress over the succeeding decades was slow. Radical changes in classification would require much more knowledge about the causes of mental disorders. Which is just what we don't have.

PSYCHIATRY AND NEUROSCIENCE

Psychiatry has bet on neuroscience as the best way to understand mental disorders, to solve problems in diagnosis, and to plan treatment. Only time will tell how this wager will pan out. Psychiatrists often claim that their field is on the verge of a great breakthrough. If one were to believe the hype, a biological explanation—and a biological cure—for mental illness lies just around the corner. (Or as one wag put it, every few years we are told that answers are just a few years away.)

Although progress in brain research has been rapid and impressive, its application to psychiatry has thus far been very limited. Brain scans are impressive—even if one keeps in mind that the colors are artificial. But all they tell you is that brain activity looks different in patients with mental disorders. The precise meaning of changes is unclear, and many are not specific to any one condition. The reality is that we do not know enough about the brain, or about the mind, to develop a truly scientific classification. And it could be 50 to 100 years before we even get close. DSM-5 needs to be written for 2013, not for 2063 or 2113.

It is understandable that psychiatry—so long the Cinderella of medicine—and desperate for respectability, wanted to plant its flag on the terrain of neuroscience. But the promise of the 1990s ("the decade of the brain") for research on mental disorders has not been fulfilled. Neuroscience has shed great light on how the brain functions, but we do not understand the etiology or the pathogenesis of the most severe mental disorders. We know that most of them are heritable but have no idea as to which (or how many) genes are involved. Although some are associated with abnormalities on brain imaging, the findings are neither specific nor explanatory. Although psychopathology is also associated with changes in neurotransmitters, the theory that chemical imbalances cause mental disorders is too simple, or plain wrong. Ultimately, it might even be impossible to fully explain mental disorders as brain disorders. The neuroscience model attempts to reduce every twisted thought to a twisted molecule. This approach devalues studying the mind on a mental level.

Considering that it will take many decades to unravel the mysteries of psychopathology, our current situation is nothing to be ashamed of. Mental phenomena reflect the activity of the human brain, which happens to be the most complex structure known in the entire universe. There are more synapses in the brain than stars in the sky.

DSM-5 need not be based on ideology and hope. The DSM-5 task force, as well as the leaders of the National Institute of Mental Health, seem to believe that psychiatry should give up its traditional mission, which was both scientific and humanistic, and redefine itself as the clinical application of neuroscience. To paraphrase a famous line from the Vietnam War, some experts want to destroy psychiatry to save it.

UNSOLVED PROBLEMS IN PSYCHIATRIC DIAGNOSIS

Lack of Knowledge about Mental Disorders: DSM-5 is not "the bible of psychiatry" but a practical manual for everyday work. Psychiatric diagnosis is primarily a way of communicating. That function is essential but pragmatic—categories of illness can be useful without necessarily being "true." The DSM system is a rough-and-ready classification that brings some degree of order to chaos. It describes categories of disorder that are poorly understood and that will be replaced with time. Moreover, current diagnoses are syndromes that mask the presence of true diseases. They are symptomatic variants of broader processes or arbitrary cut-off points on a continuum. Thus, although classifications serve a necessary function, psychiatrists can only guess about how "to carve nature at its joints." That phrase (attributed to Aristotle) describes an impossible task. We do not know if it will even be possible to find joints to be carved. Even in medicine, diagnoses are not always cleanly defined or related to a specific etiology. In contrast, mental disorders greatly overlap with each other—and with normality.

The Need for Biological Markers: In the absence of a more fundamental understanding of disease processes, DSM-5, like its predecessors, had no choice but to continue basing diagnostic criteria on signs and symptoms. But observation needs to be augmented by biological markers, as has been done in other medical specialties. In the absence of such markers, we cannot be sure that *any* category in the manual is valid. We should therefore not think of current psychiatric diagnoses as "real" in the same way as medical diseases. And listing them in DSM-5 does not make them real. For example, broad categories such as "major depression" in no way resemble diseases. Even the most "classical" concepts in psychiatry, such as the separation of schizophrenia from bipolar disorder, have not fully stood up to scrutiny. In summary, psychiatrists make diagnoses but need not reify them. They are best advised to stay humble and to avoid hubris.

Boundaries Between Mental Disorder and Normality: This is one of the most nagging problems in psychiatric diagnosis. Every edition of DSM has expanded this frontier, taking on more and more problems of living as diagnosable disorders. Psychiatric classification has become seriously over-inclusive, and the manual grows ever larger. DSM-5 errs on the side of expanding its boundaries—mainly out of fear of "missing something" or not including problems that psychiatrists treat in practice. The result is that people with normal variations in emotion, behavior, and thought can receive a psychiatric diagnosis, leading to stigma and inappropriate treatment.

Diagnostic Validity and Research: Because we have to live with a diagnostic system that is provisional—and that will almost certainly prove invalid in the long run—much of the research on mental disorders has to be taken with a grain of salt. For example, although a massive amount of data has been collected on the epidemiology of mental illness, almost all results depend on the current diagnostic system. Similarly, studies of treatment methods in psychiatry that target specific disorders are sorely limited by the problematic validity of categories. Most treatments, ranging from antidepressants to cognitive behavioral therapy, have broad effects that are not specific to any diagnosis.

Comorbidity: One of the most troubling problems with the DSM system is that it yields multiple diagnoses in the same patient. That is not the way medicine usually works. It is, of course, possible for patients to suffer from more than one disease. But in psychiatry, if you follow the rules, the same symptoms can be used to support two or three diagnoses. Thus "comorbidity" is little but an artifact of an inexact system in which criteria for disorders overlap. The sicker a patient, the more mental disorders will be identified. DSM-5 suggests severity ratings and diagnostic spectra to address this problem, but such procedures do not resolve underlying questions about boundaries.

Algorithmic Diagnosis: Another source of uncertainty is that diagnosis in psychiatry does not depend on "pathognomonic" signs and symptoms that define specific diseases. The algorithmic approach of the DSM system has been rightly popular—it uses "polythetic" criteria, making a list and then requiring a given number to be present. These quantitative thresholds are superior to asking clinicians to determine whether the patient's condition resembles a prototype. But if a typical DSM diagnosis requires, say, five of nine criteria, nobody knows whether four or six criteria would have been more or less valid. Few categories have absolute requirements for any criterion, and no system of weighting takes into account the most characteristic features. The DSM system has been jocularly called a "Chinese menu" approach to diagnosis. But most clinicians would be hard put to remember all criteria for any category.

Dimensionalization: The editors of DSM-5 suggest that the solution to the comorbidity problem is to see disorders as *dimensions*—spectra of pathology that can be scored in terms of severity. All previous editions have classified mental disorders as specific categories, much like general medicine. One of the main changes in DSM-III was the revival of that model, based on the work of the great German psychiatrist Emil Kraepelin (1856–1926). Categories are consistent with the view that psychiatry concerns itself with mental illness, not with unhappiness or life itself. They also imply that psychopathology falls into a set of "natural kinds," much like tuberculosis or many forms of cancer. DSM-5 seeks to overthrow this "neo-Kraepelinian" approach and replace it with a model in which normality and illness lie on a vast continuum. The rationale for the change is that research suggests the underlying biology of mental disorders is more dimensional than categorical. But measuring the severity of depression is not like taking blood pressure. The definition of dimensions is based on observation rather than biological markers and can therefore only be provisional. Dimensional diagnosis also runs the risk of being over-inclusive. Even normal people have some symptoms of disorder but do not deserve a formal diagnosis. If differences in degree can become differences in kind, then categories will remain necessary.

Expert Consensus: DSM-5 is not a scientific document but a product of consensus by committees of experts. Sometimes outcome depends on who gets on these committees. Where experts disagree, there is a way to "fix" the results in advance—by ensuring that membership reflects a pre-existing point of view. There are many scientific disputes affecting diagnosis, and most reflect a lack of basic knowledge. Yet as the American physician Alvan Feinstein once remarked, the consensus of experts can be the source of most medical errors.

In summary, DSM-5 is a noble attempt at a revision in line with current research and can be considered as a draft for future editions that will be based on more data. What has to be kept in mind is that the new manual only begins to develop a better framework for research and practice. Psychiatry has to put off scientifically based definitions of mental disorders to a future time when it knows more.

THE CONSTITUENCIES OF DSM-5

A diagnostic manual serves many purposes and has many potential constituencies. Let us consider each of them.

Research: Although diagnosis is an essential tool for clinical investigation, changing criteria for mental disorders leads to discontinuities, making it more difficult to compare older studies to newer ones. The question is whether changes in DSM-5 move research forward or create unnecessary confusion. Another issue is whether the more complex procedures described in DSM-5 should be reserved for researchers, who are the people most likely to apply them systematically.

Clinical Practice: The most important consumers of a diagnostic manual are mental health clinicians: psychiatrists, psychologists, social workers, and family physicians. Practitioners can use DSM on a daily basis. Researchers do not mind if procedures for reaching a diagnosis are complicated, but clinicians do. If the manual is not user-friendly, it will never be used as intended—or not used at all.

Clinicians are busy people. By and large, they do not have the time or the inclination to open a book and count criteria. (They are even less likely to score symptoms on rating scales.) That is why previous editions of DSM were never applied in a systematic way. Many (if not most) users of DSM-5 will prefer an electronic version that can be easily searched. Even so, given that previous printed editions have not been used as intended, it is unlikely that the text of DSM-5 will be regularly consulted on mobile devices.

Clinicians reach conclusions rapidly. They rarely follow algorithmic procedures and prefer to make diagnoses intuitively. Most have a prototype in their mind as to what any disorder should look like. The more closely a patient fits this model, the more likely it is that a diagnosis will be made. In this light, DSM-5 may not make as much difference to real-world practice as one might imagine. The details of DSM-III and

DSM-IV were complicated, so clinicians were happy to leave systematic diagnosis to researchers.

Previous editions of DSM were poor guides to therapy. To be fair, the system was never intended to guide treatment. (That principle was always explicitly stated, but clinicians didn't seem to believe it.) As mental health practice becomes increasingly evidence-based, it could eventually develop specific treatments for diagnoses based on research. Doing so is not possible now. Only a few well-established links are known between any diagnostic category and specific therapeutic options.

The Pharmaceutical Industry: This constituency has a strong interest in DSM-5. Companies are interested in maximizing their profits; one way to do so is to get physicians to prescribe more drugs for more people. Any change that encourages wider diagnosis of mental disorders as a whole is in their interest. Specifically, the way DSM defines schizophrenia, bipolar disorder, and major depression could have an enormous impact on industry profits. Some of the most problematic trends in modern psychiatry have resulted from attempts to make patients fit into categories that justify the prescription of drugs. The over-inclusiveness of DSM-5 should make the pharmaceutical industry happy.

The Legal System: Lawyers and judges will also be interested in DSM-5. Psychiatric diagnoses have found their way into the court system, affecting everything from criminal responsibility to custody rights and insurance payments. Although the science behind diagnosis does not justify any of these practices, they are widespread.

The General Public: Finally, DSM-5 will influence the way everyone views mental illness. Patients (and non-patients) have access to published criteria and sometimes diagnose themselves (or their relatives). This amplifies the danger that too many people will receive psychiatric diagnoses. The way consumers and families see mental problems will also have an influence on practice, most likely in the direction of more aggressive treatment.

In summary, the one certain thing about DSM-5 is that it will be another best-seller. What is less certain is whether it will lead to improved mental health care.

TEN HIGHLIGHTS OF DSM-5

Although many changes in the new manual are relatively minor, I would like to highlight areas where major revisions have been made, particularly those that have aroused controversy. All will be discussed in detail in this book.

1. DSM-5 is reorganized into a new series of chapters that either reflect common clinical features or seem to fall in the same spectrum.
2. The multi-axial system introduced in DSM-III has been eliminated. There is now no such thing as Axis II: personality disorders are considered in the same way as other categories
3. With the elimination of Axis V, levels of functioning can be rated using scores for severity or disability.
4. The criteria for several categories, particularly generalized anxiety disorder and attention-deficit hyperactivity disorder, have been expanded, which will probably lead to more frequent diagnosis.
5. The grief exclusion for diagnosis of major depression has been eliminated.
6. Substance use disorders now describe cases using the term *addiction*, and no longer distinguish between dependence and abuse.
7. Overly aggressive children can now be diagnosed as having *disruptive mood regulation disorder.*
8. *Autism spectrum disorders* now include both classical autism and Asperger's syndrome.
9. Dementias are now classified as *neurocognitive disorders,* rated by severity.
10. *Somatic symptom disorders* replace somatoform disorders and are classified rather differently.

It is worth noting, however, that some controversial changes that were proposed earlier in the DSM-5 project have been either dropped or greatly diluted. Dimensionalization has not been consistently applied, and the system remains categorical. While a major revision for personality disorder classification had been envisaged, the proposal proved overly complex, and was eventually rejected and moved to the Appendix for further study. Thus DSM-5 will revert to the DSM-IV system for these diagnoses. Also, attenuated psychosis syndrome (which might have led clinicians to treat people who have mild symptoms but never develop schizophrenia) has also been relegated to the Appendix. A proposal to reduce the length required for a hypomanic episode from 4 days to 1 or 2 was not adopted. The impact of dropping the grief exclusions in diagnosing depression has been diluted, by warning clinicians to avoid making this diagnosis when the course of mourning appears normal. The range of autism spectrum disorder has been kept limited. Finally, formal severity ratings for all diagnoses, which are too complex for clinical use, have been moved to the Appendix.

THE STRUCTURE OF THIS BOOK

The first part of this book is devoted to broader issues. Chapter 1 reviews the history of psychiatric diagnosis, Chapter 2 how diagnostic manuals are prepared, Chapter 3 how diagnoses are validated, Chapter 4 how mental disorder can be separated from normality, and Chapter 5 how dimensional assessment could be used. Chapter 6 examines clinical utility.

The second part examines the major diagnostic groups in DSM-5. Chapters 7 through 13 present separate discussions of the most frequently used diagnoses: psychoses, bipolar disorder, depressive disorders, anxiety disorders, obsessive compulsive disorder, neurodevelopmental disorders, impulse control and conduct disorders, eating disorders, sexual disorders, and personality disorders. Chapter 14 presents a briefer look at neurocognitive disorders, somatic symptom disorders, dissociative disorders, sleep–wake disorders, elimination disorders, and adjustment disorders.

In Part III, Chapter 15 examines the future of psychiatric diagnosis, suggesting guidelines for the practical use of DSM-5 in clinical work, and underlines issues that need to be resolved for the next edition—DSM-6.

ACKNOWLEDGMENTS

David Goldbloom and Ned Shorter read earlier versions of this book and provided detailed suggestions for revision. Craig Panner was an attentive and thoughtful editor. This book reflects the influence of critiques of DSM-5 published by Allen Frances.

THE INTELLIGENT CLINICIAN'S GUIDE TO DSM-5®

DIAGNOSTIC PRINCIPLES

Chapter 1

The History of Diagnosis in Psychiatry

WHY IS DIAGNOSIS IMPORTANT?

Since the dawn of medicine, diagnosis has been essential to practice. Physicians need to organize the chaos of clinical symptoms into meaningful categories of disease. They also need to make a diagnosis before prescribing treatment. Ideally, valid medical diagnoses should be rooted in an understanding of disease processes. They should be based on a specific cause (*etiology*) and on a specific pathway to illness (*pathogenesis*). Yet many categories in medicine have been little more than descriptions of signs and symptoms.

Patients come to clinical attention with physical changes (signs) and subjective complaints (symptoms). But these are only the apparent manifestations of pathology. The great advances of medicine over the course of the nineteenth and twentieth centuries depended on understanding underlying mechanisms. Some of the most important discoveries have shown that apparent symptoms (pain, fever, swelling, anemia, jaundice) can result from entirely different pathological processes.

Differential diagnosis is a "game" that every medical student is expected to learn how to play. Every set of symptoms, even the most common, can be explained by a variety of causes, and it is the job of the physician to sort out these possibilities. Differential diagnosis is much like detective work. Every detail of history, physical examination, and laboratory findings can be a clue. Arthur Conan Doyle based the character of Sherlock Holmes on one of his medical school teachers,

Joseph Bell (1837–1911), who gave his name to Bell's palsy and could deduce a great deal from a small amount of information.

The discovery of a difficult diagnosis is the subject of an even more complex game—the Clinical Pathological Conference (CPC). An expert is asked to review all the records of a difficult case, and the correct (but often missed) diagnosis is revealed by autopsy. (It has been said that pathologists are always right, but are usually too late.) These exercises have long been carried out at top medical schools, and a series has been published for several decades in the *New England Journal of Medicine*.

The detective work of diagnosis has also become the subject of popular columns in newspapers and magazines. The reader is given a clinical presentation (often from an emergency room), and the process by which an astute physician reaches a correct diagnosis is described. The main difference from a CPC is that the outcome is usually a good news story.

Despite the importance of diagnosis, physicians still spend much of their efforts treating symptoms. The great Canadian physician William Osler (1898) opposed the "shotgun" medicine of his time, in which every symptom was managed with a different drug. (As we will see, despite advances in medical science, that practice remains common, especially in psychiatry.) But psychiatry is not the only specialty in which etiology and pathogenesis are unknown. In some areas of medicine (such as infectious diseases), valid diagnoses can be based on an understanding of underlying pathological processes. In others (most chronic diseases), that is not possible.

Yet even when knowledge of disease is limited, diagnosis performs a number of important functions. First and foremost, it allows physicians to communicate with each other. When one informs a colleague that a patient has a classical case of peptic ulcer—or paranoid schizophrenia—a vast amount of information is conveyed by a single diagnostic term.

Second, diagnosis offers something important to patients: a validation that they are indeed sick, an explanation of why and what can be done for them, and a prognosis. Even when prospects for effective treatment are slim, most people feel better when they receive a diagnosis. At the very minimum, suffering is no longer a mystery, and they can expect to benefit from whatever knowledge medical science has at hand.

Third, diagnosis provides researchers with a tool for conducting investigations and for developing theoretical models of disease. That is why cancer research uses a coding of disease types and staging and why clinical research in psychiatry makes use of standardized interviews.

Fourth, diagnosis helps physicians to plan treatment and to establish a prognosis. When research is available to determine outcome, planning can be more rational.

Fifth, diagnosis aims to provide categories specific enough to guide the choice of treatment. At present, only a few treatments, such as antibiotics, can claim that kind of specificity, and even then, drugs are often prescribed without a clear idea as to what is wrong with the patient. Yet medicine is slowly but inexorably moving in the direction of specificity. Pharmacogenetics may be in its infancy but is already being applied to a few diseases. In the future, psychiatry could benefit from this approach.

DISEASES, DISORDERS, AND SYNDROMES

Valid medical diagnosis is a relatively recent phenomenon but is based on more than a century of research (Balint et al., 2006). For most of the history of medicine, illnesses could be described only as *syndromes* (a cluster of commonly associated signs and symptoms). These syndromes could have a multiplicity of causes. For example, the popular eighteenth century category of "dropsy" (swelling of the extremities) confused edema resulting from heart disease, kidney disease, and a variety of other causes. In the nineteenth century, only a few true illnesses could be properly diagnosed (mainly infectious diseases). Even so, causes were not well understood before the advent of the germ theory of disease in the 1880s, and it took many years before that theory resulted in therapeutic benefits, and before infections could be properly treated.

The late nineteenth century was a time of rapid progress in medical research. The work of chemists like Louis Pasteur (1822–1895) and of bacteriologists like Robert Koch (1843–1910) led to the identification of specific infectious agents behind many diseases. The work of pathologists such as Rudolph Virchow (1821–1902) allowed scientists to directly observe disease processes at the level of the organ and of the cell. Yet despite these advances, physicians were not yet able to help most of their patients.

By the early twentieth century, scientific medicine entered a period of ascendancy. William Osler (1849–1919) was one of the key figures. Over several decades, working at four universities (McGill, Pennsylvania, Johns Hopkins, and Cambridge), he established many of the principles that still guide medical education and practice (Osler, 1898). These include diagnosis based on detailed observation of signs, careful listening to patients' symptoms, and laboratory tests to confirm the presence of a pathological process.

As long as physicians were limited in their ability to treat disease, diagnosis did not necessarily lead to specific and effective therapy. But later in the twentieth century, medical therapeutics greatly advanced. The introduction of sulfa drugs in the 1930s and of antibiotics such as penicillin after World War II was followed by a cornucopia of effective agents for many other conditions. Then accurate diagnosis really began to make a difference. Again, the most dramatic example was infectious diseases, where lives could be saved by culturing a specific microorganism and by prescribing an antibiotic to which it was sensitive. Later, similar principles were applied to other diseases. To treat syndromes such as anemia, hypertension, and congestive heart failure, physicians need to divide them into diagnostic categories based on specific pathological mechanisms. Even in psychiatry, where mechanisms are rarely understood, bipolar disorders can be separated (at least partially) from other conditions by a relatively specific response to mood stabilizers (Goodwin & Jamison, 2007).

PRINCIPLES OF NOSOLOGY

"Nosology" refers to the science of diagnosis. This term gives the impression that diagnostic categories are scientific and based on empirical data. Yet all too often they are not.

Although the problem is more severe for psychiatry, uncertainty affects many medical diagnoses. Categories can change as knowledge increases. For example, when I was a medical student, we studied a disease called "viral hepatitis." That entity has now been subdivided into hepatitis A, hepatitis B, hepatitis C, and hepatitis D—with more to come in the future as separate infectious agents, each with a unique method of transmission, are identified. One can imagine the same process occurring in other poorly understood diseases, each of which arises from a different pathological process.

Medicine need not worry about validity for diagnoses that are based on known etiology and pathogenesis. It can also confirm many categories using medical imaging, biological markers, and cellular processes. Ideally, diagnosis evolves lock-step with research. Even so, many—if not most—diseases remain mysterious. That is particularly the case when it comes to mental disorders.

To be fair, medicine and psychiatry are not the only areas of science in which classification can be problematic. Biology offers an illustrative example. There are more than a million types of multicellular organisms, and the number of single-celled species is much larger. The taxonomy developed by the Swedish scientist Carl Linnaeus (1707–1778) was a breakthrough in its time and is still used. But as with diagnosis in medicine, classical taxonomy is based almost entirely on appearances.

Although biologists have had no trouble understanding that birds and bats belong to different groups, subtler distinctions have not always been clear. The classification of organisms can be based on evolutionary relationships, but the tools to carry out such analyses have only been available relatively recently, as the use of DNA as a marker became practical. Using this tool allowed "the tree of life" to be organized into three domains (Sapp, 2009) (Archaea, Bacteria, and Eukarya), divided into six kingdoms (Archaebacteria, Eubacteria, Protista, Fungi, Plantae, and Animalia). Even so, there are boundary problems—for example, the question as to whether viruses are living organisms.

Nuclear physics offers another example (Schumm, 2004). Matters were relatively simple when the only known particles were electrons, protons, and neutrons. As dozens of other "elementary particles" were discovered, particle physics faced a crisis. The development of quark theory resolved the problem by describing all these phenomena as combinations of much smaller entities—which seem, at least for now, to be irreducible. Even so, this classification (as well as the actual existence of some of the particles predicted by the theory) remains controversial. Although some of these problems may be resolved by experiments conducted in the Large Hadron Collider, physics, like psychiatry, may have to use a classification system that has uncertain boundaries. If the "hard sciences" face difficulties of the same kind, physicians and mental health professionals should feel a little better about their own problems in classification.

WHY PSYCHIATRIC DIAGNOSIS IS DIFFICULT

The categories used in psychiatric diagnosis are based on observation of signs and symptoms, rather than on pathological processes. One can make use of a few signs, such as facial expressions associated with depression or the flight of ideas associated with mania. But what clinicians mainly use for diagnosis are symptoms, the subjective experiences reported by patients. Psychiatrists have little knowledge of the processes that lie behind these phenomena. Thus *psychiatric diagnoses, with very few exceptions, are syndromes, not diseases.*

Many have hoped that advances in neuroscience would solve these problems. After all, changes in thought, emotion, and behavior must ultimately reflect neural processes. Disorders of the mind are also disorders of the brain. But the brain is not as easy to understand as the heart or the kidney. It may be the most complex structure in the entire universe. Thus mental disorders cannot easily be reduced to the biology of neurons. With billions of neurons, billions more glia, and trillions of synapses connecting neurons to each other, the brain does not lend itself to any simple explanation. To add to the complexity, psychological phenomena are shaped by life experiences and by a sociocultural milieu. It is not surprising that mental illness is so hard to understand.

Moreover, while mind depends on the brain, mind cannot be entirely reduced to the activity of neurons. Mental processes are "emergent" phenomena that cannot be explained on the level of cellular activity or synapses (Gold, 2009). They require another level of analysis, in which thoughts, feelings, and behaviors are studied in and of themselves.

In summary, although research has provided some insight into the localization and mechanism of brain function, psychiatry today stands about where the rest of medicine was 100 years ago. It will take many decades to answer even the most basic questions facing neuroscience. To believe that we know enough in 2013 to create a classification of mental illness based on biology is an illusion.

THE DIAGNOSTIC AND STATISTICAL MANUAL OF MENTAL DISORDERS SYSTEM

The International Classification of Diseases (ICD), a system sponsored by the World Health Organization (WHO), is the most widely recognized classification of medical illness. Even today, Diagnostic and Statistical Manual of Mental Disorders (DSM) codes are "translated" for ICD, the official worldwide system. Originally derived from a list of causes of death, the first version of ICD was compiled in 1893. Mental disorders were first listed in ICD-6, published in 1949. Although mental illnesses took time to be recognized, the WHO system has become more sophisticated with each revision, and the current version, ICD-10 (WHO, 1993) differs from DSM-IV only in detail. Currently ICD-11 is planned to appear in 2015 and to be more or less compatible with DSM-5. (It remains unclear to what extent that will be the case.)

The ICD has been eclipsed around the globe by the more detailed and systematic American system—DSM. A preference for DSM reflects the dominance of research in the United States and the wish of clinicians and investigators to use categories compatible with American science that are used in most medical and psychological journals. However, there is a more substantive reason for the greater influence of DSM. That results from the manual being *algorithmic*, so that clinicians count observed criteria and then follow an established logical sequence. This approach is, in principle, more amenable to science. It is also much easier to count criteria than to match detailed descriptions. Rather,

ICD describes *prototypes* for each of its categories, which the clinician is asked to determine if a case approximates.

This algorithmic approach to diagnosis dates from the publication of DSM-III in 1980. In 1952, the American Psychiatric Association published DSM-I, which was mainly intended to keep statistical records and was not much of a scientific instrument. I learned DSM-I as a medical student: The manual was thin, with 130 pages describing 106 disorders. It had nowhere near the impact of later editions. The most important limitation of DSM-I was that it listed disorders, described them briefly, but did not precisely define them. Without algorithms for diagnosis, reliability was inevitably low. As a result, psychiatrists could not even agree on their most basic diagnostic concepts.

For example, American psychiatrists of 50 years ago had an overly broad concept of schizophrenia and were not in accord with their British colleagues, who were more likely to diagnosis psychotic patients as having manic-depressive illness. That problem was documented by research in which videotapes of interviews were shown to psychiatrists on both sides of the Atlantic (Cooper et al., 1972). Later, American clinicians came to diagnose patients in much the same way as their British cousins.

A second problem with DSM-I was that it adhered to theoretical models that were eventually found wanting. Under the influence of the Swiss-American psychiatrist Adolf Meyer (1866–1950), who favored environmental models of etiology, almost all mental illnesses were described as "reactions." (There was even a category called "schizophrenic reaction.") Such turns of phrase imply that *all* mental disorders are reactions to environmental stressors. Although the idea contains a grain of truth, the concept is misleading. It entirely misses the essence of disease processes, which have a trajectory of their own, even when environmental factors act as precipitants. In internal medicine, stressors—both physical and psychological—can raise blood pressure, but no one would consider making a diagnosis of "hypertensive reaction."

DSM-I also reflected the strong influence of psychoanalytic theory. At that time, most of the leaders of American psychiatry were either trained analysts or sympathetic to the analytic movement.

Several disorders (mild depression, anxiety, conversions, phobias, and obsessive-compulsive symptoms) were classified as "neuroses"— a term popularized by Freud. The manual specifically stated that such symptoms were the result of "unconscious conflict." How one might assess the presence of such a process was left to the clinician. Clearly, the era of basing diagnosis on measurable phenomena had not yet arrived. In the end, DSM-I was used for hospital records but never had a defining role in research or practice. It was also not consistent with the ICD system, isolating American psychiatry from the rest of the world.

DSM-II, introduced in 1968, was taught to me when I was a psychiatric resident. Its 134 pages described 182 disorders. All these diagnoses were supposed to be compatible with ICD. The term "reaction" disappeared entirely—schizophrenia was now just "schizophrenia." However, psychoanalytic influence on the definition of disease remained in place. Neuroses were still described as resulting from unconscious conflict, as every good Freudian believed. And because the definitions of each category were not algorithmic, the reliability problem was in no way resolved.

Although all psychiatric residents had to learn DSM-II, we did not take it very seriously. For one thing, it was written in descriptive paragraphs rather than algorithmic criteria. Thus, there was too much latitude for clinicians to interpret phenomena in their own way, with the result that DSM-II diagnoses were not particularly reliable. But at the time, diagnosis had few implications for treatment. Psychotic patients were given antipsychotics, whereas antidepressants were prescribed for depression. Everyone else got psychotherapy, and diagnosis did not make that much difference in choosing how to conduct it. The classification of mental disorders only became a hot topic when DSM-III was published.

THE DSM-III REVOLUTION

In 1974, only 6 years after the publication of DSM-II, the American Psychiatric Association (APA) realized that the problems of diagnosis in psychiatry were too severe to retain the second edition. This was an era in which critics who refused to believe in the reality of mental illness were vigorously attacking psychiatry. Many had a political agenda. On the right, the American psychiatrist Thomas Szasz (1961) was a libertarian who did not want to allow any role for the state in determining personal conduct and rejected psychiatric diagnosis because it could be used to support the involuntary commitment of psychotic patients. On the left, the British psychoanalyst Ronald Laing (1967) claimed that mental illness was a response to an insane society—a point of view that fit the spirit of the 1960s. Laing was against diagnosis for the same reason he was against medication—he believed that psychosis could be a personal journey that only required an expert guide.

Obviously such critiques were well out of the mainstream of medical thought. Yet they had a wide popular appeal at the time, and psychiatry felt the pressure. Moreover, if, as research showed, diagnosis was not reliable, then no one could trust it. It was important for the field to show that the classification of mental disorders had some basis in science.

Perhaps the most important factor in the APA's decision to revise DSM was psychiatry's need to overcome its isolation from the rest of medicine (Spitzer, 1991). DSM-II was based on unproven theories and had categories that looked nothing like medical diagnoses. Thus, psychiatrists earned little respect from their colleagues. Of course, inaccurate diagnosis is not the only reason physicians disrespected psychiatry. The stigma associated with mental illness was, and remains, the most important factor (Corrigan, 2005). But the blatantly unscientific system used in DSM-II did not help.

In the course of the 1970s, the APA, under the leadership of its director, Melvin Sabshin (1902–1987), began to prepare the next edition of DSM. They chose Robert Spitzer (1932–), a professor from Columbia University, to lead the task force. This was a time of change and ferment in psychiatry, and the selection of Spitzer proved pivotal. A former analyst who had rejected Freud, Spitzer focused his career on developing better methods of assessment for mental illness.

Spitzer's concept for the new edition was based on the research of a group of psychiatrists at Washington University in St. Louis, led by Eli Robins (1922–1995) and Samuel Guze (1924–2000). These men began as renegades but became the leaders of a new psychiatry. Dismissing psychoanalysis out of hand, they wanted to move American psychiatry into consonance with traditions developed in Europe.

Spitzer was a natural ally for the Washington University group, several of whom he brought into his DSM Task Force. Like many of his contemporaries in academic psychiatry, Spitzer was disillusioned with older paradigms and looking for something different. His interest in psychometrics was based on the principle that diagnosis, as well as signs and symptoms on which categories are based, can be quantified. Spitzer was following a long-standing principle in science: The only valid concepts are those that can be measured with *numbers*.

This point of view involved a return to principles developed by the German professor Emil Kraepelin (1856–1926). Kraepelin, a contemporary of Freud, was the leading psychiatrist on the European continent in the early twentieth century and became famous for his separation of psychoses into schizophrenia and manic-depression (Kraepelin, 1921). As Shorter (1997) has observed, Kraepelin turned out to be much more important for contemporary psychiatry than Freud, whose star has rapidly faded. That is why DSM-III was described as "neo-Kraepelinian" (Klerman, 1986).

Kraepelin understood that psychiatric diagnosis must eventually be based on biological processes. But while waiting for specific markers to be discovered, categories can be provisionally based on signs and symptoms, as well as on clinical course, prognosis, and treatment response. That was precisely the view of Spitzer and of the group at Washington University.

One of the assumptions of Kraepelinian psychiatry was that categories of disease are real, even if they remain to be discovered. This view is in accord with the approach of modern medicine. Yet some see it as a form of "essentialism" that fails to acknowledge that diagnostic categories inevitably have fuzzy edges (Livesley, 2011a). DSM-5 seeks to go beyond Kraepelin, accepting categories as a temporary expedient but viewing illness as a point on a broad continuum that shades into normality.

Whether or not this paradigm ultimately prevails, in the absence of biological markers for disease, DSM-III and its successors were not in a position to reach Kraepelin's goals. But the neo-Kraepelinians rightly insisted on observable, phenomenological criteria. One of the main effects of this principle was to undermine the influence of psychoanalysis on American psychiatry (Paris, 2005, 2008a) and to replace that paradigm with a new perspective.

Some years earlier, Robins and Guze (1970) had developed a set of criteria that could be used to define schizophrenia and other major psychiatric disorders. The system focused on observable phenomena and was algorithmic (i.e., had a defined pathway from observation to diagnosis). This approach, often called the "Feighner criteria," after the lead author of the seminal paper (Feighner et al., 1972), was the germ of DSM-III. It was the model on which diagnoses in the third edition were built (Kendler et al., 2010).

The Washington University group also proposed that these "research diagnostic criteria" could be used as a general benchmark for diagnostic validity (Robins & Guze, 1970). Their idea was that all diagnoses should be based on (1) precise clinical description; (2) laboratory studies identifying biological markers; (3) clear delineation from other disorders; (4) a characteristic outcome in follow-up studies; and (5) a genetic pattern in family history studies. Although none of these criteria are directly based on etiology or pathogenesis, they could be markers for disease processes. The Robins-Guze criteria are similar to the way medical diagnoses are validated. But these goals, however modest, have proven to be beyond reach. Twenty years later, *no* major mental disorder had met this benchmark (Blashfield & Livesley, 1999), and the situation has not changed. Moreover, some of these assumptions have been challenged (Hyman, 2007). Mental disorders, if they do not correspond to strict categories, may not have the characteristic features suggested by such a paradigm.

THE IMPACT OF DSM-III

DSM-III was much larger than any previous edition: 494 pages describing 265 categories. It was a paradigm shift that threatened some, drew applause from others, and aroused great controversy. It may be hard for a new generation, brought up on this system, to understand the tumult that preceded and followed its adoption. In particular, most psychoanalysts opposed DSM-III. They rightly perceived that it contradicted their worldview and loosened their hold on the profession. Some thought the manual would destroy psychiatry. For example, early drafts of DSM eliminated the concept of neurosis entirely and made no mention whatsoever of an unconscious. For a while, angry psychoanalysts threatened to secede from APA as a group. Then, in a clever move, Spitzer fashioned a compromise in which the term "neurosis" continued to appear, but in parentheses only. (That term was dropped entirely in DSM-III-R.)

Another source of resistance was that DSM-III took, at least at first, an unfamiliar approach. Diagnosis had long been considered an art, based on clinical experience. Now, with specified criteria, anyone could do it. If you could assess signs and symptoms, then you just had to open the book and count. Making diagnosis easy demystified psychiatry, in that its procedures could be used by family doctors and by nonmedical professionals. Some thought DSM diagnosis was too robotic, but that conclusion was mistaken. A final diagnosis may depend on an algorithm, but it takes a fair amount of experience to assess whether criteria are present or whether they are clinically significant.

In the end, the momentum of DSM-III proved unstoppable. Psychiatrists were no longer willing to stand outside of medicine and be mocked and looked down on by their colleagues. Even if they could not aspire to having a specialty fully grounded in empirical data, they now had a diagnostic system that at least *looked* scientific. DSM-III met a need, and almost everyone began to use it. Today hardly anyone can remember being against it.

One of the main criticisms of psychiatric diagnosis had been that clinicians seeing the same patient might not make the same diagnosis. The absence of *reliability* was a potentially fatal problem. As every psychology student knows, measurements cannot be valid without first being reliable. Low reliability ultimately reflected the fact that the criteria sets of earlier DSM manuals were vague. If one uses a "prototype" (i.e., a description of a typical clinical presentation), then one expects the clinician to determine whether a patient's signs and symptoms approximate a written description (Berganza et al., 2005). But doing so is not easy, and different raters may still come to different conclusions. That remains the main weakness of the ICD system.

Even if you don't have the data to determine diagnostic validity, you can prioritize reliability. That is precisely what DSM-III did. The problem is that we can all agree and all be wrong. Even so, it is better to have categories on which everyone can agree. Diagnostic validity would just have to wait.

Interestingly, although some psychiatrists resisted DSM-III, clinical psychologists were generally positive. That was quite an achievement, given the traditional competitiveness between these two professions. Psychologists liked that the system looked like the criteria they learned in graduate school and used for many other purposes: relatively precise definitions, with algorithms that lead to a conclusion.

In this respect, DSM-III diverged significantly from ICD. That is why DSM took precedence—not only in the United States but all over the world. It is now difficult to find a scientific paper that does not use the DSM system or a group of clinicians for whom the manual is entirely unfamiliar.

THE DSM SYSTEM SINCE 1980

The year 1980 was a watershed. The DSM system changed relatively little over the next 30 years. It took time for practitioners to adapt to a radically new method of classification. Moreover, further changes in diagnosis could be problematic for researchers. If it was standard for all patient samples to be described according to DSM, then changing the criteria could put a research paper out of date even before it was published.

There was some tinkering in DSM-III-R (APA, 1987). The manual was now 567 pages long and described 292 diagnoses. The most significant shift was that hierarchical rules (excluding a diagnosis if another category explained the same clinical features) were greatly restricted.

That led to even greater degree of "comorbidity" (multiple diagnoses)—a problem that, as we will see, remains unresolved. Some psychiatrists felt that the changes in DSM-III-R were not sufficient to justify a new manual. Murmurings were heard that revisions were arbitrary and that they came out of informal meetings in Spitzer's basement. Suspicions were even raised about the large profits that APA made every time a revision was published.

After revolution, people crave stability. And the APA eventually decided that stability in diagnosis was more important than Robert Spitzer. To this end, it assigned a different leader: Allen Frances (1942–), then a professor at Cornell, to lead the DSM-IV process. This revision (APA, 1994) made fewer changes than DSM-III-R had. It described 297 disorders in much greater detail (886 pages!). The most major innovation was a new section on sleep disorders. Another was the publication of "source books," summaries of the research findings on which the manual was based.

At the time, Frances stated that the new manual should be good for another 15 years. He was more than right—it lasted for 19 years. Only a few minor changes were introduced in a "text revision," DSM-IV-TR (APA, 2000), which did not change the criteria for disorders but discussed them a little more thoroughly.

Only now, more than 30 years after DSM-III, is a major revision being introduced. The authors of the new manual have stated their aim to base the classification more firmly on science (Kupfer et al., 2002; Regier et al., 2009). This book will offer a critical examination of whether this goal has been reached.

Because research continues to make slow progress, it could take less than 30 years for the next major revision. The question is whether it is better to maintain stability or to introduce a system for continuous update. The reason why DSM-5 uses an Arabic (rather than a Roman) numeral is that it is open to revisions prior to DSM-6. Like computer programs that are updated on the Internet, a DSM-5.2 or 5.3 could appear sometime in the next few years. The upside is that if a great discovery is made, it can be included. Also, it may be easier for clinicians to accept change gradually. The downside, however, is that changing criteria is disruptive for both research and practice.

HOW THE DSM SYSTEM SHAPED PSYCHIATRY

Every mental health clinician will want to have a copy of DSM-5—even if they do not read it cover to cover. And the way that patients are classified will have an effect on the treatment they receive—although diagnosis does not determine therapy. Every research project in the coming years will have to take the new system into account. All diagnostic instruments based on DSM-III or DSM-IV will have to be revised. Within a few years, all medical journals receiving submissions about clinical populations will require a DSM-5 diagnosis. And the residents I teach all want to know whether they have to master the new system to pass their exams.

Textbooks of psychiatry have been built around DSM diagnoses for the last 30 years. Even doubtful diagnoses must be given their own chapter—forcing editors to choose proponents of the most controversial categories as authors. This implicit validation is one of the reasons why it has been so difficult to remove *any* diagnoses from the manual. (Even in a hard science like astronomy, the demotion of Pluto to a "dwarf planet" in 2006 drew loud protests.)

There was a time when psychiatrists were known as deep thinkers rather than classifiers of disease. All that changed in 1980. Today the field of psychiatry has come to be organized around the DSM system. It may not be, as the media sometimes claim, "psychiatry's bible." But given the general public's interest in psychiatry, each revision, including DSM-5, is important news.

DIAGNOSIS AND TREATMENT

DSM-III included a disclaimer that diagnoses based on the manual do not necessarily lead to any specific mode of treatment. However, it has been impossible to resist the linkage. Psychiatrists, as well as other physicians and clinical psychologists, are usually not interested in classification for the sake of classification. When they have a hammer, they search for nails. This can make them try to fit a patient into a category they think they know how to treat. Although today the hammer is usually a drug, diagnosis can sometimes be an attempt to fit a method of psychotherapy, as shown by the vast interest in post-traumatic stress disorder.

The pharmaceutical industry has not been shy to take advantage of these forces to encourage the use of specific diagnoses. When they market a new drug, they need to create a market for it. (These campaigns usually go under the rubric of providing "information" for practitioners.) For example, attention-deficit hyperactivity disorder is diagnosed more often now, in adults as well as in children, in part because there are new agents to replace the tried-and-true option of methylphenidate.

Similarly, one reason why major depression tends to be diagnosed is the large number of antidepressants on the market. And bipolar disorder tends to be diagnosed because of the perceived effectiveness of mood stabilizers and antipsychotics. In contrast, a relative lack of interest in anxiety disorders reflects the absence of newer and more effective pharmaceutical options.

There are exceptions to this principle. For example, there has been an increase in the diagnosis of autism and autistic spectrum disorders despite the lack of evidence for the efficacy of any therapy. Here the driving force seems to have been fascination with a diagnostic construct.

The claim that DSM-5 represents the latest in scientific knowledge is doubtful. Diagnosis is not necessarily a neutral and empirically based procedure. It is driven by a variety of social forces lying outside of medicine (Horwitz, 2002). It can be influenced by academics promoting a theory or a favorite diagnosis. It can be influenced by practitioners' desires for predictable clinical results. It can be influenced by patient advocacy—most of the main diagnoses in psychiatry now have their lobby group. It can also be influenced by the media, which have the power to affect everyone's opinion—even experts. The authors of the new manual may not acknowledge, or even be fully aware of, all these influences. That does not make them any less important.

Chapter 2

How Diagnostic Manuals Are Made

Producing a diagnostic manual is a complex process that resembles a military operation. It requires a "general" and a hierarchy of command. The American Psychiatric Association (APA) has put the creation of each new manual in the hands of a "task force" chaired by a prominent academician. For DSM-III and DSM-III-R, that person was Robert Spitzer. For DSM-IV, it was Allen Frances. For DSM-5, the role was shared between two research psychiatrists: David Kupfer and Darrel Regier.

Kupfer and Regier are prominent leaders in their field. Kupfer is a mood disorder researcher who served for 26 years as Chair of Psychiatry at the University of Pittsburgh. Regier is an epidemiologist, a research administrator at the National Institute of Mental Health, and Director of the APA's Division of Research. Their point of view on diagnosis is rooted in extensive academic and research experience. Their clinical perspective is less clear. High-ranking academics do not often see a large number of patients—many live in a rarified world that is protected from raw clinical reality. That is also true of most of the psychiatrists and social scientists working on DSM-5 committees. The experts involved in the process may therefore be influenced more by theory than practice.

The result is a manual designed to make researchers happy. Investigators have the luxury of taking all the time they need. They do not have to make diagnoses rapidly while multitasking—as many clinicians must do. Insensitivity to the needs of busy practitioners tends to make the manual unwieldy for practice. DSM-5 has worked hard to inject more "science" into psychiatric classification but may be more useful for investigators than for clinicians.

The detailed writing of a DSM manual depends on many people. The APA set up a group of task force members, most of whom were either chairs of "work groups" (each of which dealt with a major groups of disorders) or of "study groups" (each of which was asked to examine broader conceptual issues). These groups were composed of prominent researchers, and being a member was considered a great honor. The chairs were asked to choose the experts they wanted, and these decisions may well have led to predetermined outcomes.

The task force consisted of 28 people. Each of the work groups had 6 to 12 members and conducted regular meetings, either in person or electronically. (Using e-mail, they only had to travel a couple of times a year to meet face-to-face.) Their mandate was to review the existing literature, prepare new sets of criteria, and to field-test them. They were assigned to examine the following diagnostic groups: ADHD, anxiety, childhood and adolescence, eating, mood, neurocognitive, neurodevelopmental, personality, psychosis, sexual, sleep, somatic, and substance use.

The study groups were assigned broader questions. One focused on spectra that cross diagnostic boundaries, recommendations for structuring categories, and developing better overall criteria for psychiatric diagnosis. A second was assigned to look at how developmental processes influence diagnosis. A third looked at the influence of gender and culture. A fourth examined interfaces between psychiatry and medicine, with a mandate to develop a new definition of disability (to replace Axis V, the scoring system introduced in DSM-III). A fifth was assigned the task of reviewing the measurement of dimensions within categorical diagnoses.

DSM-5 conducted a series of field trials in 2011 to determine whether the system was reliable and user-friendly. This was intended to allow for fine-tuning. But, the field trials suffered from a lack of time (Jones, 2012). Also, given the lack of comparisons with DSM-IV, it was difficult to determine whether the system actually works better in practice.

There has been considerable debate in the literature about the wisdom and validity of making radical changes in a new manual. However, it was decided to begin with a new team, excluding most of the experts who worked on DSM-IV. Although the editors backed away from their initial hope for of a "paradigm shift," work groups were encouraged to be innovative. All decisions received scientific review by a separate committee of a senior academic psychiatrists. At the end of this complex process, all reports were submitted to the task force for approval. The final document of DSM-5 then had to be approved by the APA Board of Trustees in December, 2012, with the book published in time for the annual meeting in May 2013.

KEEPING INDUSTRY OUT

When DSM-III and DSM-IV were published, some critics expressed concern that the text had been subject to undue influence by the pharmaceutical industry (Kutchins & Kirk, 1997). Actually drug companies had no direct input into the DSM process. But industry benefits financially from diagnoses that lead to a wider use of products that obtain indications from the Food and Drug Administration. Also, experts in psychiatry, many of whom receive money from industry, can be biased in favor of expanding diagnostic categories. No one claims that industry can actually tell organized psychiatry how to write its diagnostic manual. But when so many of its key opinion leaders are in the pay of industry, diagnoses that lead to specific pharmaceutical indications could be more likely to get into DSM. That possibility is worrying.

Thus experts who take money from drug companies are almost bound to be biased—often without realizing that they are. They live in a climate of opinion that consistently favors new diagnoses and new drugs. That was a good reason to keep them out of the process of preparing DSM-5. But it was not possible to exclude everyone, as almost every professor of psychiatry has been supported in some way by industry. Cosgrove and Krimsky (2012) have documented how the rules were stretched in a way that reduced, but in no way eliminated, conflict of interest. The best one can say is that those who served took less. Most of them will probably go back to industry for further support once the process is over.

The APA has had a history of overly close relations with "Big Pharma." Until recently, industry sponsored many events at the annual meeting, creating profits that were used to support the organization as a whole. This led to a suspicion that drug companies could also shape DSM-5. Most industry funding is not used to support research but pays for pharmaceutical representatives and offers payment to experts who promote sales. Academics in the pay of "Big Pharma" often give talks that directly or indirectly support new drugs. They may have be paid to be "consultants" for industry or serve on "advisory boards," which usually involves little real work but allows for attendance at conferences in interesting or exotic locales. The funds that professors of psychiatry take from pharmaceutical companies have made a few of them into millionaires. The latest drugs, few of which are really different from agents already on the market, are strongly promoted by these opinion leaders, who get paid for giving talks advising clinicians to use them.

In short, it is possible for academic psychiatrists to be bought off by the pharmaceutical industry (Healy & Thase, 2003). Even one of the chairs of DSM-5, David Kupfer, has acknowledged providing services for several companies but stopped when he took on his current job. And there is little doubt that new diagnoses in psychiatry are good for business. For example, the relatively new category of social phobia generated billions in sales for the makers of antidepressants (Lane, 2007). The more categories there are in DSM-5, the better for industry.

These concerns have led to a backlash against organized medicine for its overinvolvement with Big Pharma (Angell, 2000). Despite its weak position within medicine as a whole, psychiatrists take more money from industry than any other group of specialists. These conflicts of interest have the potential to corrupt both clinical practice and research. In 2008, Senator Charles Grassley of Iowa brought these issues to public attention. The spotlight was placed on academic psychiatrists taking millions of dollars from industry in "consultant fees" for promoting products in lecture tours. As reported in the New York Times (June 8, 2008), the chair of psychiatry at Emory University lost his job when these facts came out and when it became clear that he had not informed his university or the NIMH about how much money he had been paid. (This psychiatrist had no trouble getting another chairmanship because of his fame and a close relationship to the leaders of NIMH.)

New guidelines governing the relationship between industry and professional organizations in medicine have been proposed to deal with these problems (Rothman et al., 2009). The DSM-5 process required that all task force and work group members be vetted and that only minimal involvement with pharmaceutical companies would be allowed from the time of participation. This rule slowed down the entire process (it took a full year to vet everyone). In the end, all task force members were declared to be "clean" of major involvement with industry. But if almost all of them have taken money from pharmaceutical companies in the past, one cannot be certain whether their objectivity is permanently compromised.

TRANSPARENCY VERSUS SECRECY

The process of preparing DSM-5 has been criticized for insufficient transparency (Frances, 2009a, 2009b, 2009c). A document with such an enormous influence on practice cannot be prepared in secret and needs to have a degree of "buy-in" from potential users. Although all proposals for change were eventually put on a website for commentary, the initial process by which the new manual was revised was far from open.

The authors of earlier editions took greater pains to consult widely. For years before the publication of DSM-III, I remember well-attended symposia at each annual meeting of APA in which all changes were discussed and feedback seriously considered. (I even wrote Spitzer with a question, and got a typed reply.) When DSM-IV was being prepared, drafts were sent for comments to experts who were not members of the work groups. (I was one, even if my comments had little effect on the outcome.) In contrast, the DSM-5 process was, at least at first, closed. This created suspicion that the task force wanted to avoid criticism, and hoped to present psychiatry with a *fait accompli*.

In a spirited exchange published in the newsletter *Psychiatric Times*, Frances (2009a, 2009b), joined by Spitzer (2009), criticized a confidentiality agreement signed by all work group members. Everyone had to promise to keep discussions under wraps. This rule threatened to close the whole process to feedback. Both Frances and Spitzer also suggested that because many of the revisions under consideration were problematic, they needed to be openly and intensively debated outside the task force.

A group representing DSM-5, led by a president of APA (Schatzberg et al., 2009), wrote back to deny these claims. They argued that early drafts were too provisional to be up for general discussion and noted that the most major changes were being presented at a number of scientific meetings. Unfortunately, this letter included a nasty counter-accusation, raising serious questions about the judgment of those who wrote it. Schatzberg et al. claimed that the authors of previous editions (i.e., Frances and Spitzer) were motivated by a financial interest in books and assessment measures they published after DSM-III and DSM-IV. This comment made no sense, because nobody will buy these books once DSM-5 is in place. (Schatzberg himself had been accused of conflict of interest by Senator Grassley for promoting drugs in which he had a financial interest.) The tone of this reply shows how badly APA was stung by criticism.

The process of writing the manual should have been more open from the beginning. When you are making changes that may or may not be valid or user-friendly, you should circulate proposals widely and open them up to scientific debate. The bigger the decision, the more input from clinicians and researchers is needed. Although everyone eventually had the opportunity to submit suggestions on the Web, I doubt that they were taken seriously.

In the end, all proposed changes were published on the DSM-5 website in February 2010. Further revisions were posted in 2011 and 2012. One suspects that this happened as a result of criticism and pressure from higher levels, which created a new committee in 2009 to oversee the entire process (chaired by a former APA President, Carolyn Robinowitz).

Frances and Spitzer (2009) also complained that no one outside the committees had access to the data driving the revision. In DSM-IV, the driving principle was that any changes must be justified by evidence. That evidence was summarized in a four-volume "sourcebook" (Widiger, Frances, & Pincus, 1997), put out a few years after the revision itself. There are no plans to publish a similar document for DSM-5. Rather, one can consult the website, in which changes are explained and justified with reference to the scientific literature. However, when these preliminary reports from the work groups were posted in February 2010, they only offered brief rationales, not detailed literature reviews, data analyses, or critical comments about criteria. This vagueness suggested that some of the revisions were based on opinion rather than data, as has happened in previous editions (Lane, 2007). Being vague deflects comment and prevents researchers not on the task forces from making informed critiques. Moreover, proposals were not sent to potential opponents to avoid bias, as had been the policy in DSM-IV (First, 2010). Finally, the document as a whole was not presented to experts entirely outside the DSM-5 process for independent assessment. Because peer review is a basic principle in science, DSM-5 risks being *less* scientific than its predecessors.

Many academics only had their first good look at the proposed changes in February 2010. By the time the DSM-5 website opened, the process was well advanced, and workgroups had been meeting for 2 years. Although a few changes were made after that, the train had already left the station.

Perhaps the real problem lies not in process but in the fact that DSM-5 is more driven by ideology than any previous manual. The guiding principles are that mental disorders are neurobiological and dimensional and lack a cut-off from normality (Kupfer & Regier, 2011). The agenda is to overthrow the neo-Kraepelinian paradigm. But as of 2013, the data are not there to support such a change. DSM-5 cannot be a paradigm shift, and those who originally thought so could be guilty of hubris.

Even so, we need to understand the point of view of the new manual. Some changes can indeed be rationalized by empirical findings. But DSM-5 often lacks clinical utility. The academics who wrote it may not have slaved away, like most of us, in a clinic or emergency room for years but spent much of their careers in front of computer screens. That is why they have not given the proper weight to clinical practice. This circle might have been squared if DSM-5 had been published in two versions: one for daily clinical use and one for research. That idea has been supported by some commentators (McNally, 2011) and seems sensible. But for the APA, dividing DSM-5 in two has no traction, because doing so would be seen as compromising its scientific cachet.

In the end, DSM-5 has made the same mistake one sees in many decisions made by governments or corporations. Without criticism from outsiders, "groupthink" takes over (Janis, 1972). We have often seen this happen in political decision making, ranging from the Bay of Pigs to the invasion of Iraq. From my own knowledge of colleagues who served on the work groups, I think some signed on to changes they didn't believe in to achieve a consensus.

A CAUTIONARY TALE

One of the most serious omissions in the process of creating a new manual is the absence of any direct comparisons between DSM-IV and DSM-5, accompanied by an assessment of the clinical and research impact of changes. The omission was deliberate, because the editors saw DSM-IV as invalid and did not see any value in head-to-head comparisons. Moreover, the task force made a point of *not* consulting either Frances, the editor of DSM-IV, or Spitzer, the editor of DSM-III. Many other senior figures in psychiatry were left out of the loop. Leaving experts out of a process, and not even asking their opinion, was unwise. It led in some cases to open opposition (both through the scientific literature and the public media). The feeling of the leadership was that the time had come for radical change and that although outsiders might disagree with changes, they would eventually have to come around, as they did after DSM-III. But there was a price to be paid.

The DSM-5 process downplayed continuity (First, 2010). The most radical proposed revision was for personality disorders, a diagnostic group seen as ripe for dimensionalization. This story turned out to be an epic of hubris and downfall. Although some degree of change was warranted, the proposed revision was unwieldy and problematic (see Chapter 13).

I was one of those left out of the revision process, but my criticisms, which mainly had to do with poor clinical utility, were not based on personal pique. The opinion of *most* senior investigators in my area was never formally solicited. Anyone with views that contradicted the agenda was either not heard or written off as a dinosaur. The result was that experts not included turned against the proposals, albeit for different reasons. Thus, every time the new criteria were presented at conferences, they were heavily attacked by researchers not included in the process. Opponents, even as their suggestions were rejected, were forced to write articles in journals and/or letters of protest to the APA. The only way to exert influence on the process was informal, through personal relationships with work group members. I wrote some work group members and organized a group for a conference call with the chair of the personality disorder work group, but had little influence on the outcome. But there were serious differences between members of the work group, some of whom were strong supporter of dimensionalization (Livesley, 2010), while others defended categorical diagnosis (Shedler et al., 2010). Still other experts (e.g., Frances, 2010d) suggested leaving things more or less as they are until more evidence becomes available.

In the end, the personality disorder proposal was rejected by the Board of Trustees on the advice of its scientific advisors. It went too far beyond empirical data, and was considered as "a bridge too far." This was not the best way to prepare a diagnostic manual that will shape clinical work and research for many years to come.

TIMELINE

One of the most searching criticisms of the DSM-5 process concerned its tight timeline. Although planning started many years ago, time ran out faster than expected (as it always does). The outcome reflected what could be called a "rush to judgment."

Anyone who has seriously studied psychological assessment knows that measurement of psychopathology is a complex and slippery business. It can take years to establish validity for the simplest scale, whether based on self-report or on clinical assessment. How then did DSM-5 introduce new and relatively untested ways of assessing psychopathology in such a short time? The process tells us more about politics than about science.

Jane Costello is a researcher at Duke University who has made important contributions to the new field of developmental epidemiology (the study of mental illness in the community over the life span). Costello had been appointed to the work group on child and adolescent disorders but left in the summer of 2009, posting her resignation letter on the Web. Costello (2009) raised several problems about the DSM-5 process. She did not agree with rewriting the entire manual at one time, as opposed to doing so piecemeal as data came in. As Costello remarked, "I am not aware of any other branch of medicine that does anything like this." Costello's comment on the timeline was, "…as time has gone by, the gap between what we need to know in order to make revisions and what we do know has grown wider and wider, while the time to fill these gaps is shrinking rapidly. More and more, changes seem to be made for reasons that have little basis in new scientific findings or organized clinical or epidemiological studies.…I continue to be shocked that the APA would even consider revising the DSM without being willing to allocate the funding necessary to carry out the underlying scientific studies. A drug company that tried to bring a product to market on the basis of inadequately-funded research would rightly be censured."

Costello concluded that the APA needed to spend more money and time on research. For example, concerning the decision to dimensionalize some DSM-5 criteria, she asked, "on what grounds, anyone with any experience of instrument development knows that what they proposed last month is a huge task, and a very expensive one. The possibility of doing a psychometrically careful and responsible job given the time and resources available is remote, while to do anything less is irresponsible."

From a scientific point of view, Costello was perfectly right. If categories are not valid, then no amount of finessing can correct the problem. But DSM-5 is *not* a scientific instrument. The APA's priority was for a new manual, published on time (even if, in the end, it wasn't). A book that is used by every mental health professional cannot be easily revised piecemeal. A manual that stays on the bookshelves of clinicians for years has to be reasonably stable, even when it is wrong.

Another reason why DSM could not be delayed is that the APA was short of funds. That situation resulted, in part, from a backlash against corruption by the pharmaceutical industry. For many years, the annual meeting of APA was supported by industry-sponsored symposia. Under pressure from politicians and journalists, the APA and industry have agreed to go their separate ways (and the annual meeting is now a day shorter). But if budgets had to be cut back, then DSM-5 could not be readily extended beyond the extra year that put it off to 2013. Or to wait till 2015, the year that ICD-11 will come out.

Although everyone agreed the system needs to be fixed, the editors of DSM-5 were given a rare opportunity to revolutionize psychiatry, which they took as a mandate. The idea that most things should be left alone until we know more was not on their agenda.

Did the pressure to complete a revision in a short time make the outcome worse? Or was this just the best that could be done under the circumstances? This book will offer many criticisms of the task force decisions. But I am not sure whether taking more time would have made a difference. Here is the reason. Although DSM-IV wasn't good enough, we didn't have the scientific knowledge to improve on it. Literature reviews and field trials conducted by work group experts can only produce, at best, educated guesses.

Despite all the criticisms I have raised, psychiatry cannot stand still. After 33 years with the same system, it needed to try something else. If we wait until all the data are in, then we could wait for decades, while stuck with a problematic classfication. So DSM-5, even if it is no better than DSM-IV, still had to be written. And although some changes are ill-advised, some are indeed an improvement.

In the end, the ambition of the editors was too great, producing an outcome that was not a great improvement over its admittedly defective predecessors. Unfortunately, this is not an abstract scientific dispute. Getting diagnosis wrong has consequences. The classification system used in psychiatry has real effects on real patients. If the categories are wrong, too many people will receive the wrong diagnosis and the wrong treatment.

Moreover, once a system is in place, it is carved in stone for years to come. Whatever the problems, no one will want to change the manual again soon. If major revisions are not introduced for another 15 years, some of us may not live that long. So we are stuck with a flawed system that that will affect practice for most of our professional lives. We have to use DSM-5 but need to work our way around it. This can be done if we keep in mind that diagnosis in psychiatry is a tool for communication, that categories are not yet as real as medical illnesses, and that classification is bound to change over time as new data comes in.

FIELD TRIALS

To determine whether new diagnostic methods are feasible and valid, one needs to conduct *field trials.* These procedures involve testing new procedures on suitable patient populations, determining reliability and clinical utility. On the positive side, samples were generally large, and fairly representative of practice, and ratings were done by clinicians, rather than researchers. However, these trials only began in 2011, leaving little or no time for fine-tuning or replication.

More extensive field trials would have held up DSM-5 for a few more years, although no serious harm would have been done by the delay. Conducting these trials under a tight deadline was a recipe for trouble. That, and a lack of funds, made the trials inadequate. One cannot introduce new and complex measures without much more time and trouble. The results may or may not be generalizable, At best, the field trials provided a ballpark estimate for reliability but don't tell us much about validity or clinical utility.

Medical research, like all science, requires replication (ideally with sufficient data to conduct a meta-analysis). Samples have to be representative, and replications crucially important. Diagnostic procedures need to be tested on real patients (not video simulations, as in some trials) and carried out in large numbers at multiple sites. DSM-5 worked on another principle: ready or not, here we come! That is why results from the DSM-5 field trials may not reflect the real world of practice, where clinicians have to make diagnoses rapidly, without having time to ponder over precise criteria.

The results of field trials can, to some extent, be determined in advance. You can run almost any system past raters and come up with reasonable reliability—after a bit of training. Meanwhile validity remains a distant dream. Again, because there was no direct comparison to DSM-IV in the field trials, the process sheds little light on whether DSM-5 is any better than its predecessor. Although the editors of DSM-5 believed they were applying principles that are better based in theory, researchers, even after the DSM-5 criteria were posted, have not yet examined the effects of the new system on case identification and prevalence in clinical and community samples.

In the end, DSM-5 repeated some the mistakes of its predecessors. The field trials for DSM-III and DSM-IV had also been rushed and failed to include replication procedures. And for many disorders, reliability was only marginally acceptable. Surprisingly, nobody paid much attention to these numbers, which are not better in DSM-5. In fact, reliabilities of 0.5 were deemed "acceptable" by a group of epidemiologists associated with the DSM-5 project (Kraemer et al., 2012). It is hard to believe that experts reached conclusions that would not be accepted in most journals. The best one can say about the field trials is that they suggest that DSM-5's procedures can be followed by clinicians when treating real patients.

HOW DIAGNOSTIC MANUALS ARE USED

Neither DSM-I nor DSM-II were best-sellers. The manuals gathered dust on shelves unless used for statistics. But with the advent of DSM-III, every psychiatrist, clinical psychologist, psychiatric social worker, psychiatric nurse, and mental health researcher *had* to look at the manual. The readership also included lawyers and judges. And patients themselves, particularly since the advent of the Internet, began to look up their diagnoses and to read the criteria on their own.

Few formal studies have shown how clinicians use the DSM manual in daily practice. Ideally, one should read criteria carefully before making a diagnosis. (Nobody can remember them all.) Algorithims are supposed to be followed with precision, but that doesn't actually happen (Zimmerman & Galiano, 2010). Clinicians retain a general idea of the criteria for a disorder if they have made a diagnosis before. They rarely stop to count criteria. And many incorrectly rely on one or two criteria (the ones they remember) to make a diagnosis. The manual is more likely to be opened if a clinician sees a patient with symptoms that are unfamiliar and do not correspond to a well-known prototype. In that case, DSM may provide some degree of help.

The situation is different in research. Investigators assess subjects using diagnoses based on DSM criteria, although that is not good enough for publication in many medical journals. Editors and peer reviewers know that the reliability of clinical diagnosis is not high, so diagnosis by structured interviews is usually expected (Miller et al., 2001). But these methods of clinical assessment, however reliable, are ultimately based on the manual, so they do not make DSM categories any more valid.

Lawyers have a different agenda for DSM. In criminal cases, a defense attorney may try to use diagnosis to get a client off a charge. Under the classic "McNaghten rule," you have to show that a defendant could not distinguish right from wrong at the time he or she committed the crime, (i.e., to have been psychotic). For example, the DSM-III criteria for schizophrenia became part of the evidence in the famous trial of John Hinckley, and the diagnosis was the subject of cross-examination in court. (There was even testimony about Hinckley's abnormal brain scan.)

Similarly, lawyers in civil cases may introduce evidence based on DSM categories. I have been threatened a few times with subpoenas in child custody cases, asked to give testimony about diagnoses that could be made on one parent or another. That assumes, incorrectly, that one can predict parenting capacity from a psychiatric diagnosis.

Even historians have been interested in the DSM manual, retrospectively diagnosing famous people according to its criteria. (More frequently, these diagnosticians have been psychiatrists who are amateur historians.) This has led to absurd claims, like calling Winston Churchill "bipolar." Although physicians outside psychiatry have also fallen into this trap, applying a category of mental illness to a long-dead person is fraught with problems. Perhaps the exercise aims to validate psychiatry and reduce stigma by showing that famous people have had mental disorders. But it only succeeds in making diagnosis look ridiculous.

To take a recent example, every great eccentric in history may be seen to have suffered from autism or Asperger's syndrome (James,

2006). One of the candidates, Albert Einstein, was peculiar but had two wives and many mistresses—hardly the picture of an autism spectrum disorder. Similarly, the claim that artistic geniuses (such as Robert Schumann) had bipolar disorder (Worten, 2007) ignores the well-known fact that syphilis (called by physicians "the great imitator") was highly prevalent throughout the nineteenth century and that Schumann died after falling ill suddenly and spending a year in a mental hospital. Without a blood test for *treponema pallidum*, it is idle to speculate about the dead.

Living people may be interested in their psychiatric diagnosis, whether or not they have ever seen a mental health professional. Patients and their families benefit from the ready availability of DSM criteria for common categories of mental disorder. And if they haven't done so, I tell them to look them up. Yet in my experience, patients get into the same trouble as clinicians in going from signs and symptoms to diagnosis. They focus on one feature from which they may draw wide conclusions. Most people think in a linear fashion—understanding complexity is a skill that has to be painfully learned. By and large, nonlinear thinking (i.e., seeing the development of illness in terms of multiple pathways and multiple outcomes) is more common among researchers, and even there one may look for it in vain.

ADDING DIAGNOSES

Each time the DSM comes up for revision, lobby groups organize to influence the outcome. Sometimes their goal is to drop a diagnosis entirely. (I supported a group that advocated the elimination of dissociative disorders in DSM-5—which, as discussed in Chapter 14, did not happen.) More often, the aim is to introduce a new diagnosis or group of diagnoses that clinicians or researchers consider important. When a new edition is about to come out, you can expect someone to promote a pet category.

Many suggestions concern pieces of the clinical puzzle not currently considered as disorders. Some are not based on theory or research but on the need to make clinical work reimbursable by insurance. Consider, for example, a proposal to include a category of "relational disorders" (First et al., 2002). That diagnostic group was defined as "persistent and painful patterns of feelings, behaviors, and perceptions among two or more people in an important personal relationship, such a husband and wife, or a parent and children." The main reason for introducing this group would be to allow couple and family therapy to have a diagnostic code. That kind of therapy does not fall within a medical model.

Yet *most* people have marital or parenting problems of *some* kind, which does not mean they should receive a diagnosis. If mental health professionals choose to treat relational problems, then they are practicing clinical psychology but not medicine and should charge for their services (and accept the risk of not being paid by insurance). The practice of psychotherapy leaves plenty of scope for evidence-based treatment of established psychiatric diagnoses. Fortunately, DSM-5 did not adopt this proposal.

Anyone can write a set of criteria that follow the format established in DSM-III. You only have to define a diagnosis and write a list of criteria. Just add water and mix! The result can *look* as scientific as anything else in the manual. Deeper questions about the validity of these proposals can only be answered by research.

IS DSM-5 MORE SCIENTIFIC?

In promoting DSM-5 as "more scientific" than its predecessors (Kupfer & Regier, 2011), APA puts great emphasis on psychiatric research over the last 20 years. One cannot deny there has been real progress. (As one of the thousands of contributors to that literature, I wouldn't want to think I have been wasting all my time and energy!) But that doesn't mean that we know enough to diagnose patients scientifically. Unfortunately we tend to lose sight of the fact that progress in research is a small drop in a very large bucket. We know so little about mental illness. Psychiatry is a century behind the rest of medicine.

This situation is far from unique in science. Consider, for example, the enormous gap between a profound understanding of DNA and protein synthesis versus a very limited knowledge about the construction of complex biological structures. Or, consider the gap between the Big Bang theory and the structure of matter and the universe. Isaac Newton, a truly revolutionary thinker in science, once described his contribution in this way: "I was like a boy playing on the seashore, and diverting myself now and then finding a smoother pebble or a prettier shell than ordinary, whilst the great ocean of truth lay undiscovered before me."

The idea that science has progressed rapidly enough to make diagnosis more scientific may have stimulated a proposal by Insel et al. (2010). This visionary idea suggests that the National Institute of Mental Health should support studies of "research domain criteria" (RDoCs), rather than categorical diagnoses (which often do not yield consistent findings in research). It offers a matrix in which broad spectra, Negative Valence Systems, Positive Valence Systems, Cognitive Systems, Systems for Social Processes, and Arousal/Regulatory Systems, are matched with data based on genes, molecules, cells, neural circuits, physiology, behaviors, and self-report. The value of this model remains unproven, but it is fully consonant with the approach of DSM-5. And like the new manual, it assumes a level of knowledge that lies far in the future. Researchers with humility should understand they are part of a great chain of investigation that will take decades, if not centuries, to accomplish. DSM-5 is different, but the science needed to support its ideology does not yet exist.

THE STRUCTURE OF DSM-5

DSM-5 is divided into three sections: Section I is an introduction, Section II a list of diagnoses with criteria, and Section III an Appendix of proposals requiring further study.

Hundreds of diagnoses have been listed in every version of the DSM manual. But much as species fall within larger groups of orders and kingdoms, mental disorders can be classified into chapters. A "meta-structure" of this kind for DSM-5 was published in 2011. The chapters are reasonably familiar but have a few controversial elements, related to the ideology of the new manual. And despite favoring broad spectra of illness, DSM-5 has 20 chapters. (This book will generally follow that system.)

The main change is that disorders beginning in childhood are no longer considered as separate, because many continue into adulthood and because many adult disorders have childhood precursors. Thus neurodevelopmental disorders include several conditions beginning in childhood that continue into adult life: intellectual developmental disorders, language developmental disorders, autism spectrum disorder, attention deficit hyperactivity disorder, learning disorders, and motor disorders. Disruptive, impulse control, and conduct disorders all describe categories previously classified separately because they begin in childhood but usually have consequences in adulthood.

The other chapters are more familiar. Schizophrenia spectrum and other psychotic disorders is a traditional and coherent grouping. Bipolar and related disorders also include classical illnesses, although their range remains controversial. Depressive disorders comprise another clear grouping, although their homogeneity is controversial. Anxiety disorders is now a narrower group than in DSM-IV, now limited to panic, phobia, social anxiety, and generalized anxiety disorder, and there are separate chapters for obsessive-compulsive and related disorders and for trauma and stressor-related disorders.

Other chapters describe dissociative disorders, somatic symptom disorders, feeding and eating disorders, elimination disorders, and sleep–wake disorders. Sexual disorders are divided into dysfunctions, gender dysphoria disorders, and paraphilias. Substance use and addictive disorders also include some types of behavioral addiction. A chapter on neurocognitive disorders replaces the older categories of delerium, dementia, and amnestic syndrome. Personality disorders constitute a separate chapter, but Axis II has been eliminated.

After splitting these logs, there are still quite a few chips lying around—some of which fall into a chapter called "other." Although the chapters generally make sense, one still has the impression that the deck has been shuffled but the cards remain the same.

RISK, BENEFIT, AND CHANGE

If you believe that science always advances, then you could see every new edition of DSM as reflecting the march of progress. Yet every change carries a risk–benefit ratio. Most changes in DSM-5 are being presented as benefits without risks. Experience with previous editions suggests otherwise.

The main risk is overdiagnosis, and the result of overdiagnosis is usually overtreatment. We will see many examples of these problems later in this book, as we examine major depression, bipolar spectrum disorders, attention deficit hyperactivity disorder, and many other categories. Moreover, as the next chapter will show, psychiatric disorders have no clear boundary with normality. But with ever-widening criteria for diagnosis, more and more people will fall within its net. The result is that many will receive medications they do not need.

A question might be raised as to whether resistance to changing the manuals represents "conservatism." The answer is yes, but science is—and *should* be—intrinsically conservative. Change should not be based not on hope but on hard data. Although one sometimes sees true paradigm shifts, most research in science progresses incrementally (Kuhn, 1970). Conservatism is also justified by the fact that the majority of scientific papers are never replicated (Ioannidis, 2005). That is why evidence-based medicine must often wait for sufficient data to conduct meta-analyses and why treatment guidelines such as Cochrane reports and NICE guidelines are famously cautious.

In summary, despite all the defects in DSM-IV, psychiatry must hesitate to make radical changes unless the evidence for doing so is clear, not to say overwhelming. It is better to put up with a familiar, albeit flawed, system than to make unjustified changes. As Kendler and First (2010) have argued, when you don't know enough, gradual and iterative change is better than a paradigm shift. We need not leap out of the trenches into a diagnostic no-man's land. It makes sense to be patient and retain most aspects of the current system until we have enough data to change it in a valid fashion.

Although DSM-5 is not radically different from DSM-IV, this problem has run through every edition of the manual. DSM diagnoses have often failed to be conservative about separating mental disorders from problems in living. Yet earlier editions were more cautious, listing conditions that almost everyone would agree are true illnesses. But after DSM-III, and with each subsequent revision, the scope of psychiatric diagnosis expanded. One can readily reject critiques from anti-psychiatrists that DSM wants to make everyone "crazy" (Kutchins & Kirk, 1997). But the categories of DSM are definitely over-inclusive, and some are not even valid outside Western culture (Watters, 2010). Although there can be little doubt about the validity of severe mental disorders, many categories in the manual skirt on the edge of normality. The medicalization of ordinary life has sometimes been called "psychiatric imperialism" (Moncrieff, 1997). In the name of science, that is what much of DSM-5 promotes.

Chapter 3

What Is (and Is Not)
a Mental Disorder

One of the most serious problems for DSM-5 is that it extends the concept of mental disorder. It can be used to diagnose those who only have subclinical symptoms or problems. This danger is associated with the creation of new categories as well as with broader definitions of existing ones.

We need to decide what we mean by "mental disorder" and to differentiate it from life's vicissitudes—what Freud (1896/1957) once referred to as "normal human unhappiness." This definition is crucial for determining the scope of psychiatry (McNally, 2011; Kagan, 2012). The ultimate question is whether DSM-5 describes a set of illnesses or problems associated with living in the world.

DISEASE AND DISORDER

Medicine describes pathological states with terms such as *disease* or *illness*. Disease refers to physical abnormalities (such as anatomical lesions, physiological, or biochemical changes) that cause discomfort or dysfunction. Illness is often used as a synonym for disease but may also be used to describe the subjective feeling of "being ill" (Eisenberg, 1977).

In psychiatry the use of the term *mental disorder* reflects the problem in defining true diseases of the mind. A disease process is based on a known and specific etiology and pathogenesis. But there are no consistent biological markers in psychiatry reflecting the pathological mechanisms behind mental illness. This was so 40 years ago (Kendell, 1975) and remains so today (Paris, 2008a). Thus clinicians have to rely on signs and symptoms that cause distress or disability. But psychiatrists may forget that disorder is not disease.

Finally, although the use of the term "mental disorder" is less potentially stigmatic than "mental illness," some clinicians and patients still try to avoid it, in favor of misleading and vague concepts such as "mental health condition." But whatever you call them, mental disorders are frightening and threatening to personal autonomy, so their stigma can be reduced but not eliminated.

DEFINING MENTAL DISORDER

DSM-5 offers a complex definition of mental disorder. Patients must have a behavioral or psychological syndrome or pattern that reflects an underlying psychobiological dysfunction, the consequences of which are clinically significant distress (e.g., a painful symptom) or disability (i.e., impairment in one or more important areas of functioning), that must not be merely an expectable response to common stressors and losses (e.g., the loss of a loved one), a culturally sanctioned response to a particular event (e.g., trance states in religious rituals), or a result of social deviance or conflicts with society. A disorder should have diagnostic validity based on a set of external validators (prognostic significance, psychobiological disruption, response to treatment), and clinical utility (contributing to better conceptualization, or to better assessment and treatment). Finally, diagnostic validators and clinical utility should help differentiate the disorder from its "near neighbors."

As in all editions since DSM-III, the definition of mental disorder includes a set of caveats. Thus, symptoms must not appear as a part of normal development or reflect cultural variations alone. They must not be developmental quirks (such as the moodiness of normal adolescents) or cultural patterns (such as the possession states cultivated by some religions).

Each category in the manual needs to meet this overall definition. But because pathology and normality can sometimes lie on a spectrum, psychiatry should be conservative about decisions to change criteria or to add or delete any category. Given that even minor changes in wording can vastly increase the prevalence of a diagnosis, a risk–benefit analysis could have been applied to assess the impact of any changes from DSM-IV to DSM-5. We need to be sure that benefits follow from changes. Yet over the years the DSM system has been more notable for adding than for subtracting, even when additions carry an unknown risk.

THE THEORETICAL AGENDA OF DSM-5

Traditionally, medicine has defined disease in a way that separates pathology from normality. We all suffer illness from time to time but otherwise consider ourselves as normal. Psychiatry took the same view for most of its history, and it remains reasonable to separate disease-like disorders such as schizophrenia, bipolar disorder, and melancholic depression from reaction patterns like mild depressive or anxiety disorders. The neo-Kraepelinian model of mental disorder was in accord with these principles. But practitioners want a system that covers all conditions they are asked to treat, and some clinicians see people who are more unhappy than ill.

Psychiatry is not alone in this regard. Medical theory and practice has been gradually expanding its scope, "medicalizing" subclinical symptoms as well as life's ups and downs. For example, people can go to doctors to adjust their cholesterol level, in the absence of any symptoms of disease. It has been suggested that this trend suits pharmaceutical companies, who engage in "disease-mongering" to increase profits (Moynihan et al., 2002).

DSM-5 seeks to overturn the neo-Kraepelinian model and replace it with one in which illness is not separate from normality but defined by a cut-off point on a continuum. Kupfer and Regier (2011) have suggested that diagnostic spectra are supported by neuroscience research. This implies that even if people feel normal, everyone may have a bit of mental illness. It has long been known that mental disorders lack a sharp separation from normal functioning—or from each other (Kendell,

1975). But once we identify mental disorder in everyone, the concept loses meaning, and the scope of psychiatry becomes overly broad.

THE BOUNDARY BETWEEN ILLNESS AND LIFE

An old witticism states that life is a disease, for which psychiatry is the cure. Behind the joke lies a reality: It is not obvious what distinguishes mental disorder from unhappiness. Psychiatry distinguishes between sadness and depression, between moodiness and bipolarity, and between eccentricity and psychosis. That is what has traditionally defined the very concept of psychopathology.

The DSM manuals suffer from what military historians call *mission creep*, a gradual but inevitable expansion of a mission beyond its original goals. As Horwitz (2002) pointed out, the distinction between severe mental disorders and milder disorders that reflect distress in the face of circumstance has often been ignored. Many categories are included that do not meet overall criteria for a mental disorder, in that they present symptoms that produce distress but are reactive rather than innate. But DSM has been written to include every sort of problem, whether or not it constitutes a disorder. This undermines the validity of the entire system.

Because no one can say what is or is not a mental disorder, all editions of DSM have suffered from over-inclusiveness. Thus "medicalization" reformulates the human condition as a set of illnesses—that is, problems that lie beyond one's personal control (Conrad, 2007). Medicalization often comes not from physicians but from patient groups seeking to destigmatize problems. Thus, Alcoholics Anonymous promoted a medical model of problem drinking long before physicians accepted it. Similarly, consumer groups have actively promoted diagnoses such as attention-deficit hyperactivity disorder (ADHD) and post-traumatic stress disorder.

Almost everything that creates trouble in human life can be found in the DSM manuals. Badly misbehaving children can be diagnosed with conduct disorder (Wakefield et al., 2002). Adults who are painfully shy can be diagnosed with a social anxiety disorder

(Horwitz & Wakefield, 2012). Low feelings after personal losses may justify a diagnosis of depression (Horwitz & Wakefield, 2007). Recurrent episodes of rage can be diagnosed as intermittent explosive disorder. It does not even matter how common the problem is—even tobacco addiction is listed as a mental disorder.

Given this level of inclusiveness, it should be not surprising that epidemiological studies, such as the National Comorbidity Survey (NCS-R), which examine the community prevalence of DSM-defined disorders, have found mental disorders to be very common. About 20% of the population will meet criteria for at least one disorder in any given year, and at least half will do so in a lifetime (Kessler et al., 2005a). Some have argued that even these numbers are too low. Moffitt et al. (2009), reporting on a prospective community study of a sample followed from childhood to age 32 years, found that prevalence of disorders measured at the time they actually appear was nearly *double* than what people remembered and reported in retrospective studies.

Evidently mental disorder is ubiquitous. But if the lifetime prevalence of physical illness is 100%, then 50% for mental disorders would be an encouragingly *low* number. However, there are other explanations for these epidemiological findings. When prevalence is very high, you have to ask whether measurements are accurate. All these numbers assume the validity of the categories listed in the DSM manual. That is a very big assumption. In the first large-scale survey, the Epidemiological Catchment Area Study (Robins & Regier, 1991), estimates were much more cautious. But since then, diagnostic inflation, based on expansion of many DSM categories, has led to much higher prevalence estimates. It is also possible that psychiatric epidemiology has made a fundamental error by agreeing to measure DSM categories, rather than the symptoms on which they are based.

One also needs to be sure that a disorder is disabling in some way. This principle led DSM-IV to require all diagnoses to be based on symptoms that are *clinically significant*. That concept requires a serious judgment call. In major depression, Wakefield et al. (2010) argued that if symptoms already measure subjective distress, adding this requirement does not distinguish cases from non-cases. The real question concerns severity. What is the cut-off point at which distress and disability qualify as mental illness?

Many problems that merit a diagnosis under the current system are painful but not disabling. For example, mass screening methods for depression are more likely to uncover transient episodes than clinical conditions that could benefit from treatment (Thombs et al., 2008; Patten, 2008). Thus, even if most people who meet criteria for psychiatric diagnoses are never treated (Kessler et al., 2005b), that need not be a matter of great concern, as long as the sickest patients find a pathway to care.

Psychiatry is a branch of medicine, but one does not expect the majority of the population to have either clinical or subclinical disorders of the heart, kidney, or liver. This is what makes the findings of epidemiological research based on DSM categories hard to swallow. One might say that a prevalence of 50% reflects a reality we just have to accept. In fact, the leaders of the National Comorbidity Study, a large-scale epidemiological survey based on DSM-IV (Kessler et al., 2005a), have taken the view that psychiatry, like the rest of medicine, must make room for mild and subclinical disorders in its classification system. Much as general physicians treat common colds as well as pneumonia, mental health clinicians need not actively discourage people with less severe problems from coming for help. Kessler et al. also argued that mild disorders could be precursors of more severe disorders at some later point—in which case, early treatment might be preventive. However, they did not provide data on how often that happens or whether prevention is a practical option.

Admitting subclinical phenomena into a diagnostic classification is a very slippery slope. The lifetime prevalence of mental disorders could easily come to approach 100%. The boundary between normality and pathology would be completely lost. Unless disorders are defined in a way that requires real dysfunction, almost every bump on the road of life will be considered pathological. These problems also follow from the view that psychopathology of all kinds is dimensional and lies on a spectrum with normality (Pierre, 2010). Thus everyone has a mental disorder, the only question being how much. This paradigm threatens to trivialize psychiatry. To be taken seriously, psychiatry has to define disorder in a way that recognizes a difference between problems of living and illness.

HARMFUL DYSFUNCTION

Jerome Wakefield, a professor of social work at New York University, is a seminal figure in the debate about the boundaries between normality and pathology. He has proposed defining mental disorder in terms of a construct he calls *harmful dysfunction* (Wakefield, 1992).

These are two words, each of which requires a precise definition. For Wakefield, dysfunction refers to an inability to carry out life tasks specified by evolutionary mechanisms. Thus conditions like psychosis, melancholic depression, or severe substance abuse prevent people from looking after themselves or from living in families and raising children. In severe mental illness, dysfunction is obvious because it leads to striking disability. The problem lies with boundary cases. At what point is reduced function considered dysfunction? The word "harmful" adds a component of values. It means that symptoms hurt those who suffer them and/or other people with whom they are involved. But nearly every symptom patients experience is harmful in *some* way.

The usefulness of Wakefield's definition is that to define disorder, *both* harm and dysfunction are required. Thus, behavior that is only harmful (e.g., laziness, rudeness) would not justify a medical diagnosis. Nor would behavior that is only dysfunctional (e.g., drunkenness). A hybrid definition, combining harm and dysfunction, aims to cut this Gordian knot. Even so, determining whether each of these criteria is present requires judgment calls that may not be strictly objective, and there is an overlap between harm and dysfunction. The definition of mental disorder in DSM-5 is not very different from the concept of harmful dysfunction, but the devil lies in the details.

THE SCOPE OF DSM

Mission creep has steadily expanded the boundaries of mental illness. If a survey examining the presence of mental disorder identifies people who consider themselves normal, but who actually meet criteria for a diagnosis, then that constitutes a *false–negative*. But if the same survey identifies people as having a disorder when criteria are not met, then that constitutes a *false–positive*. The concept of mental disorder used by the DSM system is most likely to lead to false–positives. This problem bedevils DSM-5. It has no way to separate clinical from subclinical phenomena. And it is up to the clinician to decide what is "significant." In the absence of a precise definition, the concept of clinical significance can only be imprecise.

Since the third edition, DSM has included an increasingly long list of diagnoses. Every edition since has grown larger in scope, and the size of the manual has also grown. Again "mission creep" rules. Observing this trend, Zorumski (2009, p. xxvi) commented wryly:

> "…. one might conclude that either the field has advanced greatly or we have now generated a system that codifies many poorly studied and poorly validated descriptors."

Spitzer once told me he wrote DSM-III with the aim of being "inclusive"—he thought it best to include more categories and sort out their validity later. That was a mistake. What Spitzer did not take into account is that once a category is listed in the manual, it is very hard to remove. Too many people have a stake in maintaining it. When it came time to publish DSM-IV, only a few diagnoses were taken out, whereas many others were added.

DSM-5 has also failed to remove invalid diagnoses. But, to its credit, it did not accept every proposal for new diagnoses. One example is the category of "relationship disorder" (First et al., 2002). Problems with other people, without overt symptoms, are ubiquitous and do not constitute a mental illness. Many reasonably normal people get divorced, never marry, or fail to get along with their children. A serious potential for mission creep is driven by the fact that insurance companies expect DSM categories to be coded to reimburse clinicians. But although people who are unhappy with their relationships (sometimes called "the worried well") may seek psychotherapy, they do not have a medical diagnosis. If DSM had agreed to include relationship disorders, then psychiatry could have congratulated itself on finally succeeding in raising the prevalence of mental disorder to 100%.

Yet DSM is already sufficiently elastic that people with very mild symptoms can be diagnosed with *something*. As shown in a survey of patients in psychoanalysis (Doidge et al., 2002), many patients who are functional enough to afford this expensive treatment meet criteria for common mental disorders (anxiety and mood disorders). Some also meet overall criteria for a personality disorder, although there is a difference between lifelong dysfunction with a wide range of problems and only not being able to relate to an intimate partner. Quite a few people who seek therapy hold steady jobs and have relationships (even if they are not fully satisfactory). These people are troubled but not ill. DSM allows for the possibility that a patient can have no mental disorder but still have problems that are a focus of treatment. These problems can receive "V codes" (meaning that the patient has life problems but not mental disorder). Insurance does not pay for the treatment of such cases.

To avoid mission creep, DSM should have confined itself to problems that almost anyone would call a mental illness. This could be accomplished by reducing the number of categories and/or by making severity criteria more stringent. Then we might truly have a manual of mental disorders, rather than a classification of life.

SENSITIVITY AND SPECIFICITY

Every psychiatric diagnosis is a trade-off. *Sensitivity* measures the proportion of positive cases correctly identified. *Specificity* measures the proportion of negative cases correctly identified. Every time you widen the criteria for any diagnosis, although you may succeed in finding cases that might have been missed, you run the risk of diagnosing people who are *not* cases.

DSM, from the very beginning, has lacked specificity, resulting in multiple diagnoses ("comorbidity"). Moreover, there have been more diagnoses in each edition, and criteria have tended to soften over time, with more unhappy people seen as depressed, more moody people considered to be bipolar, and more inattentive people considered to have ADHD. DSM-5 moves even further in the same direction, loosening up the criteria for many disorders. That result is what one should expect from work groups filled with academic mavens. Experts usually believe that the disorders that most interest them are more prevalent than anyone realizes, even if they masquerade as other problems. The inevitable result is that more and more people are defined as ill.

MENTAL ILLNESS AND STIGMA

Much more than any physical illness, mental illness is associated with stigma (Corrigan, 2005). Despite all the progress psychiatry has made, the situation has not changed much. Stigma reflects negative social judgments about people who suffer from psychological problems of any kind. Perhaps these attitudes derive from the fear we all have of being out of control of our own minds, leading to a critical view of mental illness and the mentally ill.

Stigma reflects the way we think about ourselves. Life is rarely easy, even for those who think of themselves as mentally healthy. When upsetting things happen, such as the loss of a job or a relationship, it is normal to experience psychological symptoms. It is not helpful to label these reactions with a diagnosis. Actually, people benefit from normalizing such experiences. Periods of low or anxious mood can be seen as a "rough patch" rather than an illness. And although nobody feels stigmatized by a common cold, receiving a diagnosis such as depression can have real negative effects. Similarly, what is the benefit of diagnostic labeling for common problems ranging from social awkwardness to the benign loss of memory that most people experience with age?

DSM-5 should have maintained a boundary between true illness and life's bumpy road. But influenced by the principle of dimensionality, it chose not to do so. Ironically, the view that we are all a little ill was held by Sigmund Freud and was long a principle of psychoanalysis—the theory overthrown by DSM-III. Neurobiological models of mental disorder have brought us full circle.

DIAGNOSIS IN CHILDHOOD

DSM-5 is designed for patients of all ages and makes a point of not separating adult and child psychiatry. This is a good idea, because so many disorders begin in childhood and continue into adulthood. But children do not always come to clinical attention, unless parents and teachers are worried about them. Moreover, most patients seen in child psychiatry are boys, in contrast to the female predominance in adult psychiatry. The reason is that boys are more likely to have externalizing disorders that create trouble for others, which is what usually motivates a referral.

Some mental disorders are dormant in childhood and only emerge in adulthood, and many symptoms begin in adolescence (Copeland et al., 2009). We often do not know whether diagnoses made in childhood are early forms of an adult disorder, separate disorders, or a bump on a developmental pathway. To answer this question, we need long-term follow-up research. Psychiatry has few studies of this kind, largely because prospective research is so expensive. The patients seen in child psychiatry do not always come back as adults, and many of the adults psychiatrists see were never patients as children. Only a few categories (severe ADHD and conduct disorder) are known to show developmental continuity. A complex picture has emerged, in which some forms of pathology improve with age, whereas others are precursors for serious problems later. We are only at the beginning of the research that could address such questions.

It is difficult to determine the community prevalence of mental disorders in children and adolescents (Roberts et al., 1998). Much information has to be gleaned from interviewing parents. When researchers try to determine how many children meet criteria for *any* DSM category, results tend to be inconsistent. The British are generally more conservative about diagnosis, and one survey in the United Kingdom (Ford et al., 2003) found an overall prevalence of diagnosable disorders of 9.5% in a community population of children. In contrast, a community survey of children in an American rural area from ages 9 years to 13 years (Costello et al., 2003) found that 31% of girls and 42% of boys met criteria for at least one DSM-IV disorder. These numbers need to be questioned. They depend on the validity of information, the choice of cut-off points for dysfunction, and the vagaries of DSM definitions. Using a more stringent cut-off for severity, Costello et al. (2005) found that about one-fourth of those met diagnostic criteria in a year, more similar to what one sees in adults (Kessler et al., 2005). That is still a very high number. These complications raise questions about the scope of diagnosis in child psychiatry. The underlying problem is similar to what we have seen in adults—what is a disorder, what is a time-limited problem, and what is a normal variant?

Rutter (2011), a senior British child psychiatrist who has always been dubious about the validity of psychiatric diagnoses, commented in detail on the directions being taken by DSM-5 and ICD-11 in children and has made a number of provocative but useful recommendations:

1. There are far too many diagnoses, leading to a high rate of supposed comorbidity. If the number were drastically reduced, then so would the overlap between diagnoses.
2. There is no need for a separate grouping of disorders with an onset specific to childhood. Rather, the various specific disorders being placed in appropriate places in a classification that cuts across all developmental stages. (DSM-5 has adopted this change.)
3. A group should be formed of disorders known to occur but for which further testing for their validity is needed. This would allow new categories to be tested before being reified and cast in stone. (This is the function of the Appendix to the manual.)
4. Categorical and dimensional approaches to diagnosis can be combined. However, dimensions should only be introduced where there is good evidence to support them.
5. The requirement of impairment should be removed from all diagnostic criteria, given problems in reliability and validity. Rather, functioning should be coded separately.
6. Research and clinical classifications should be kept separate. (That would have been one of my own recommendations for DSM-5.) Doing so would make clinical utility much easier to achieve. Similarly, there is a need to develop a primary care classification for both medical and non-medical primary care.

Each of Rutter's suggestions leads to a more conservative, evidence-based approach to psychiatric diagnosis. They also have implications that go far beyond child psychiatry and address problems that afflict the DSM system as a whole. I can only state my approval and my regret that most of these sensible principles were not adopted

DSM-5 AND THE ROLE OF THE SPECIALIST

DSM-5 has many purposes. If it were to concentrate on being a scientific categorization of mental illness, then it would be less inclusive. When every human problem finds a place in the diagnostic manual, psychiatry's mission to provide specialized medical care to severely ill people is undermined.

When psychiatry moved back into the medical mainstream, it returned to its historical roots and to the treatment of severely ill patients (Paris, 2008a). The focus of practice has greatly changed. Psychiatrists now define themselves by their expertise in psychopharmacology, backed up by diagnostic acumen. Most now spend little time on psychotherapy which in the future may not be carried out by medical specialists. Psychotherapy for psychiatrists could become like physiotherapy for orthopedic surgeons—a procedure to be referred out to another clinician. The role of the psychiatrist now focuses on patients who need their unique skills, rather than on those who could be managed by other mental health professionals.

Psychiatrists play a crucial role as consultants. They are trained to evaluate pathology and to establish a diagnosis. DSM-5 should support this priority, not undermine it. That is another reason why it needs to distinguish between patients who have illness and who need medical treatment from those who can see other professionals for life problems. Although psychiatrists still need to know how to carry out psychotherapy, they should not offer it to normal people, even if the DSM system has categories that could justify doing so. At the same time, psychiatrists are prescribing vast amounts of medication to relieve unhappiness and common human problems. As Sartorius (2011), one of the prime movers behind ICD-11, has warned, psychiatry could lose public respect if its classification conflates mental illness with normal experience.

Yet in all fairness, psychiatry is only doing what the rest of medicine has been doing for some time—overdiagnosing patients who are not ill but who have risk factors for illness and treating people who may not need treatment. One only has to look at the history of medicine's approach to cholesterol levels or hypertension to find examples. Moreover, early diagnosis has become such a priority that people without a disease are being treated as if they had one. And the case of blood tests for prostate cancer shows that even biological markers provide no protection from overdiagnosis and overtreatment.

DIAGNOSTIC INFLATION AND DIAGNOSTIC EPIDEMICS

Failing to draw boundaries between pathology and normality leads to *diagnostic inflation* (Frances, 2009c). There have been several examples in recent years, with increasing identification of conditions such as bipolar disorder, ADHD, autism, and generalized anxiety disorder (GAD). Each of these diagnoses has a fuzzy boundary with normality—bipolarity could just be moodiness, ADHD could just be impulsivity or inattentiveness, autism could just be social ineptness, and GAD could just be a tendency to worry too much. But the DSM system has encouraged physicians to identify all these conditions as mental disorders. This has probably led to an enormous number of false–positives.

In some cases, the increase in identification has been so dramatic that one can speak of a *diagnostic epidemic*. Conditions that once seemed rare have now become common. No one seems to be able to escape the possibility that being different will be labeled as being disordered. The problem of false–positives in diagnosis is encouraged by a system that is more concerned about "missing" something than about giving incorrect labels and unnecessary treatment to normal people. The consequences can sometimes be severe. If moody people are called bipolar, then they will be treated with drugs that can have dangerous side effects. If impulsive or inattentive people are routinely diagnosed with ADHD, then they may be put on stimulants for years. If socially awkward people are called autistic, they will suffer unneeded stigma. If worried people are diagnosed with GAD, then they will be put on antidepressants that may or may not be helpful. Similarly, the interest in identifying mental disorders even before they start has created another set of problems. If one is too quick to diagnose early psychosis, or neurocognitive disorder, then patients who will never develop a serious mental disorder will be stigmatized and treated unnecessarily.

The diagnostic categories in DSM, which are at best provisional, are unavoidably fuzzy, blending into normality at the edges. But through constant usage, clinicians have come to think of them as valid, in the same way as pneumonia. Thus diagnoses in psychiatry easily become "reified"—hypothetical constructs treated as if they were real. We forget that categories are only a way of communicating. We can only await the day when we truly understand mental illness, but in the meantime, we should be careful about making diagnoses too easily. It takes time to know what patients are really like, some diagnoses are made "on the fly" by practitioners who are too busy to take the necessary time. Although psychiatrists need a classification system to talk to each other, and to patients and families, in a shared language, they have sometimes used diagnosis to describe life itself.

Chapter 4

Diagnostic Validity

"Validity" refers to whether an instrument accurately assesses what it sets out to measure. Validity is an essential element of medical diagnosis. Valid diagnoses should not be the creations of enthusiastic clinicians, but be based on empirical data and multiple indicators. As in medicine, psychiatric diagnoses need support that is independent of clinical observation, and biological markers should eventually become a crucial element in making them. But currently, validity is only a long-term goal. Even the most modest proposals are unattainable ideals. The reason is that not enough is known about the causes and nature of mental disorders. Most categories in DSM are syndromes of uncertain validity. Some, particularly the psychoses, have more data behind them than others. But even categories as widely used as major depression, or attention deficit hyperactivity disorder, reflect more about expert consensus than science. And consensus is based on compromise, not fact.

RELIABILITY AND VALIDITY

As every psychology student is taught, reliability comes before validity. Measurements cannot be reliable unless raters agree on them—at least most of the time. In principle, reliability has been supported by DSM's algorithmic procedures. Clinicians are guided to a conclusion by criteria rooted in clinical observation and asked to count how many of them are present. But getting observers to agree on whether specific symptoms are present or absent, or whether they are clinically significant, is not simple. Some are obvious (delusions and hallucinations). Others are subtle (mood instability and impulsive behavior patterns).

Although the reliability of diagnosis in psychiatry is better than it was prior to 1980, it is far from satisfactory. In the field trials of DSM-III, reliability was not very high. The standard is a statistic called *kappa*: "fair" if kappa lies between .41 and .60; "good" between 60 and 74; whereas excellent is 75 or higher. But even for a category as basic as major depression, reliability is only fair to good (Keller et al., 1995). In the DSM-5 field trials, reliabilities were low, particularly for major depression (Regier et al., 2013). Clinicians are not generally aware of this problem. If they did, they would be less likely to believe that psychiatric diagnoses are written in stone.

The reliability problem was not solved by the field trials for DSM-5. Even if kappas were as good (or as bad) as in previous editions, there is no assurance that they translate into reliability in the real world of clinical practice. Moreover, field trials are only a first step. Worryingly, the task force suggested that 0.5 is "good enough" reliability for DSM-5 (Kraemer et al., 2012). These authors pointed out that any medical diagnoses based entirely on clinical observation do no better than that. However, psychiatry, which does not have access to confirming laboratory tests, needs to set the bar higher, rather than lower.

Why is reliability so problematic and where do the problems lie? In a large sample of outpatients, Brown et al. (2001) reported on what produced disagreement in the diagnosis of anxiety and mood disorders. The issue was not so much the presence or absence of clinical symptoms. Rather, reliability was compromised by "boundary problems"—that is, determining whether symptoms are *clinically significant*. At what point can we say that a symptom causes dysfunction or is disabling? This is why boundary problems bedevil most diagnostic procedures in psychiatry. They are linked to the question of what is, and what isn't, a mental disorder.

Another problem affecting reliability is widespread comorbidity. The term "comorbidity" is a confusing misnomer that implies that a patient has two or more disorders. The overlap we see in practice might be more usefully called "co-occurrence." Multiple diagnoses are an artefact of a system structured to produce them. Given that so many categories have overlapping criteria, this result is inevitable. High levels of comorbidity, as in anxiety and mood disorders, could suggest that disorders arise from a common matrix (Goldberg & Goodyer, 2005). And most of the time, diagnosis of more than one disorder adds little to our understanding, so clinicians choose the one they consider most important.

A few diagnoses are genuinely comorbid. The best example occurs when substance abuse complicates a mood disorder. In such cases, making two diagnoses is logical because addiction has its own trajectory and requires separate treatment (Compton et al., 2007). With this in mind, clinicians correctly speak of patients with drug and alcohol problems as having a "dual diagnosis."

CRITERIA FOR VALIDITY

The criteria for validity in psychology and medicine have been defined in various ways but can be boiled down to a few basic concepts (Strauss & Smith, 2009). *Descriptive validity* (whether methods of measurement are accurate) is the most fundamental principle. *Face validity* (whether a measure seems, on the face of it, to describe a phenomenon) is not so useful, as indirect measures can be as good as, if not better than, criteria that seem intuitively "right." *Predictive validity* (whether a measure predicts outcomes such as clinical course or treatment response) is particularly important.

The type of predictive validity that psychological assessment has always emphasized is *construct validity*—that is, whether internal measures correlate with external measures. In other words, you need to show that different methods of assessment come to the same conclusion. Cronbach and Meehl (1951), in one of the most highly cited papers in the history of psychology, applied this principle to psychological testing. Construct validity is equally important for diagnosis.

These principles were the basis of the well-known Robins and Guze (1970) criteria for valid diagnosis. These authors described five criteria that are still invoked, largely because they place psychiatry in the same frame as internal medicine. The first precise, clinical description is the basis of the DSM system. Signs and symptoms need to be observable, with features that can be described reliably. Immeasurable concepts (such as mental conflict, as in DSM-II) are discarded. Thus the spirit of the DSM system eschews armchair theories of any kind. Even so, clinical descriptions do not always produce reliable measurement and therefore fail to shed light on validity.

DSM-5 has suggested quantifying these fuzzy clinical descriptions though scoring procedures. In the words of the nineteenth century British physicist Lord Kelvin (1889), "when you can measure what you are speaking about, and express it in numbers, you know something about it; but when you cannot measure it, when you cannot express it in numbers, your knowledge is of a meager and unsatisfactory kind." Even so, it remains to be seen whether scores based on clinical observation can improve diagnostic validity.

The second Robins-Guze criterion was another form of construct validity: laboratory studies to identify biological markers. When physicians observe jaundice, and liver function tests are also abnormal, they have an independent source of validity. This possibility is alluded to in the DSM-5 definition of mental disorder. Unfortunately, biological markers remain unknown in psychiatry, so this source of validity remains out of reach.

The third Robins-Guze criterion is clear delineation from other disorders. In this respect, the DSM system has been a notable failure: overlap is the rule, not the exception. Disorders frequently co-occur, and a decision to remove hierarchical rules for diagnosis in DSM-III-R only made the situation worse. The idea was that if no one knows which one is primary and which is secondary, the presence of one diagnosis should not exclude another. In practice, very few patients can be described by a single category. But massive comorbidity reflects a serious lack of validity in the entire system. In a widely quoted article, Kendell and Jablensky (2003) suggested diagnosticians should look for "zones of rarity" between disorders. But no one has, thus far, been able to find them—not for severe disorders like schizophrenia or bipolar disorder, nor for common problems like depression and anxiety.

The fourth Robins-Guze criterion is another form of construct validity: a characteristic outcome in follow-up studies. Kraepelin (1921) distinguished schizophrenia from bipolar illness on this basis (schizophrenia tends to deteriorate without full remission, whereas bipolar disorder tends to be intermittent). Yet such distinctions are far from absolute. More and more evidence has been accumulating pointing to overlap between the major psychoses (McDonald, 2004). Severity of illness may be a better predictor of outcome than categorical diagnosis.

The fifth Robins-Guze criterion, another source of construct validity, is a genetic pattern in family history studies. Family history is an indicator of heritability that can be much more easily measured than genes. But up to now, this line of investigation has not been very fruitful. What seems to run in families are not categories but broader dimensions of psychopathology—tendencies to psychosis, to moodiness, or to impulsive behavior. Because these diagnostic spectra are not confined to single categories, they undermine the validity of a neo-Kraepelinian system.

In summary, after 40 years, the Robins-Guze criteria remain visionary; we are in no position to apply them, and they could even be wrong. It could be 50 years or 100 years before we know enough to reach a final conclusion. Meanwhile, DSM-5 has taken a different approach, downplaying neo-Kraepelinian assumptions in favor of a dimensional neurobiological model.

SEMI-STRUCTURED INTERVIEWS AND SELF-REPORT MEASURES

Clinicians rely on observation to make diagnoses. Yet there are ways to make the assessment of signs and symptoms more precise. One can try to ensure that everyone is observing the same thing. For example, although interviewing is a skill, not every interviewer can be counted on to ask the same questions. Clinicians go about things in their own way and rarely use the DSM in a systematic way.

That is the reason for the development of a series of *semi-structured interviews*, whose content is defined by specified areas of inquiry that must be covered. (The "semi" part means that raters can ask questions naturally, in their own words, rather than follow a script). Semi-structured interviews became a cottage industry after the publication of DSM-III. They have the potential to make diagnosis more reliable (Garb, 2005; Mullins-Sweatt & Widiger, 2009), but not all interviews are created equal. Some of the most widely used instruments are directly derived from DSM criteria and follow them closely. What these measures ensure is that all key questions are asked, so that sufficient information has been collected to rate criteria (Rettew et al., 2009). If DSM definitions are not gold standards, then this approach is obviously limited. Thus validity is ultimately no better and no worse than DSM categories.

The best-known instrument has been the Structured Clinical Interview for DSM Disorders (SCID): the SCID-I for Axis I, supplemented by the SCID-II for Axis II (Spitzer et al., 1992). Developed for DSM-III, these interviews replaced a Schedule for Affective Disorders and Schizophrenia (SADS; Endicott & Spitzer, 1978), based on "Research Diagnostic Criteria" developed by the group at Washington University. The SCIDs were revised as the manual itself went through several revisions, and reliability studies were conducted on the DSM-III-R version (Williams et al., 1992). (We will need a new set for DSM-5.) The K-SADS, a widely used interview in child psychiatry, also follows DSM-IV criteria (Hersen, 2003). Semi-structured diagnostic interviews that are not based on the DSM system apply similar principles. The Present State Examination (Wing, 2009), originally designed for epidemiological studies by the World Health Organization, is based on ICD criteria. It has been used in Europe for both clinical and research purposes.

Some interviews are designed for specific disorders. At times, researchers have developed a measure because DSM is seen as deficient. The broader the diagnosis, the more likely it is to lack specificity and overlap with other categories. For example, in borderline personality disorder, the Diagnostic Interview for Borderlines, Revised (DIB-R; Zanarini et al., 1989) defines this category more narrowly (and more precisely) than DSM-IV.

The problem is that anyone that wants to develop an interview can do so—and give it an acronym that carries a scientific gloss. In one case, researchers studying the dubious group of dissociative disorders (*see* Chapter 14) were interested in appropriating the "SCID" brand, and convinced Spitzer to allow them to call an instrument the "SCID-D" (Steinberg & Hall, 1997). The association with a standard acronym gave the impression that this measure was empirically grounded. But all it did was to guide clinicians to apply the DSM criteria when interviewing patients.

Semi-structured interviews are valuable tools in research. Few journal articles are published today that do not use them. But their application requires training, which is why research papers usually have to report inter-rater reliability. Given the time to administer them, and the need to train clinicians in their use, these instruments are not suitable for practice.

There are also clinician-administered ratings, such as the Brief Psychiatric Rating Scale (BPRS; Overall & Gorman, 1962) and the Clinical Global Impression (CGI; Guy, 1976). These scales have been widely used in research (Leucht et al., 2005), and because they are simple to score, are sometimes applied in clinical settings. The most widely used measures are the Hamilton Scales for anxiety and depression (HAM-A; Hamilton, 1960; HAM-D; Hamilton, 1959). Even after 50 years, these scales retain a niche. They should be revised (the HAM-D is heavily loaded with insomnia questions) but have been used for so long and are so familiar that nobody wants to give them up. Moreover, checklists are easy to score and only take a few minutes of clinician time.

Psychiatry has always emphasized interviewing skills but useful information can also be gleaned by administering self-report questionnaires. The Symptom Check List, 90 (SCL-90-R; Derogaitis, 1975) is one of the most widely used general measures of psychopathology. The Beck Depression Inventory (BDI; Beck et al., 1996) is a popular self-report measure used to score the intensity of depression. There is also a widely used self-report measure for alcoholism: the Michigan Alcohol Screening Test (MAST; Shields et al., 2007). These measures do not need training to establish inter-rater reliability, as is the case for interviews. The problem is that self-reports do not always measure the same phenomena that clinicians are interested in.

Self-report measures are particularly useful in research, as they are standardized, and because subjects will only put up with a limited number of interviews. Clinicians need not use them, because most of the same information can be obtained in a few minutes of evaluation. Although questionnaires could be administered in a waiting room, they would require time for scoring and interpretation. Clinicians, therefore, are perfectly right to continue to depend on their own interviews to make diagnoses. The main role of self-report instruments and semi-structured interviews is in research studies, where one has to be sure that different observers are measuring the same thing. Checklists are no substitute, however, for the clinical diagnosis of mental disorders.

EFFECTS OF AGE, GENDER, AND CULTURE

DSM-5 has expressed interest in taking into account the effects of age, gender, and culture on diagnosis. To this end, it set up work groups to examine these issues. All these factors can have an effect on the validity of diagnosis: if disorders present differently at different ages, differently in men than in women, or differently in one culture than in another (Narrow et al., 2007).

Age: Although DSM-5 has avoided defining a separate group of childhood disorders, psychopathology often presents differently early in life than it does after puberty. For example, children are rarely psychotic, although they can develop symptoms that are precursors to psychotic illness later in life (Erlenmeyer-Kirling et al., 2000). It used to be thought that children do not develop clinical depression either, but they do—they just do not talk about feelings in the same way as adults (Cytryn & McKew, 1996). Other diagnoses, such as antisocial personality disorder or attention-deficit hyperactivity disorder, clearly start in childhood and are made in adults who have not remitted from earlier symptoms.

By and large, the earlier the onset of a mental disorder, the more severe and chronic will be its course (Paris, 1999). That is because temperamental, rather than environmental, factors are predominant in early-onset disorders. This principle is most clearly established for diagnoses that first appear in childhood, such as disruptive behavior disorders. Severe patterns of misbehavior can meet criteria for conduct disorder (CD). But when CD begins in the preschool years, the syndrome is most likely to continue into adulthood as antisocial personality disorder (Zoccolillo et al., 1992). On the other hand, when problems begin only in adolescence, they usually remit by young adulthood (Moffitt, 1993).

Most clinically important mental disorders begin after puberty. There is also a relationship between onset and prognosis. In schizophrenia, early onset is associated with a poor outcome, as well as cognitive deficits and negative symptoms (Engqvist & Rydelius, 2008; Rajii et al., 2009). In bipolar disorder, an early onset is associated with severity and chronicity (Perlis et al., 2009). An early onset of unipolar depression also predicts a more chronic course (Coryell et al., 2009).

Adolescence is also a common age of onset for anxiety disorders, substance abuse, eating disorders, and personality disorders. This may reflect hormonal changes that influence how mental symptoms develop. Another explanation could be that brain circuits are pruned and modified during adolescence. Another possibility is that the psychological challenges of this stage are stressors in vulnerable adolescents.

When a disorder begins later in development, prognosis tends to be better, because some life tasks will already have been successfully carried out. A young adult who has never worked and has not finished an education will have more difficulty recovering from mental symptoms than a middle-aged person who is established in life. Moreover, the disorder itself may look different. For example, there are not as many negative symptoms following an episode of late-onset schizophrenia (Gottesman et al., 1982).

Yet these distinctions are not always consistent. For example, although DSM-III stated that schizophrenia cannot be diagnosed if the first onset comes after age 45 years, later research showed that late-onset cases are clinically indistinguishable from early-onset cases (Gottesman, 1992). In the absence of markers to explain why the process begins in late middle age, the restriction was dropped in DSM-IV and has not reappeared in DSM-5. By and large, age of onset is more useful in determining prognosis than in defining disorders.

Gender: It has long been known that many mental disorders vary in prevalence between males and females (Narrow et al., 2007). For example, schizophrenia is somewhat more frequent in men (Thorup et al., 2007). In bipolar disorder, overall prevalence is equal, although men tend to have an earlier onset (Kennedy et al., 2005). In major depression, a 2:1 or 3:1 ratio in favor of women is seen all over the world, a finding that has been much discussed and is still in search of an explanation

PART I DIAGNOSTIC PRINCIPLES

(Culbertson, 1997); it is unlikely that these differences are entirely cultural (Weissman & Klerman, 1985). But severe depression in men is associated with a higher suicide rate in almost all countries, whereas women attempt more but use less lethal means (Beautrais, 2001).

The tendency for depression to be more frequent in females is open to several interpretations. It might reflect social disadvantage, hormonal influences specific to women, or genetic predispositions that differentially affect the genders. It is possible that all three factors play a role. However, because gender differences are seen in many different cultures, their effects on prevalence are unlikely to result from social disadvantage alone (Weissman & Klerman, 1985).

Alcoholism and substance use disorders are a mirror image of depression, in that in all countries where surveys have been conducted, ratios strongly favor men (Wilsnack et al., 2009). But women can be addicted to other behaviors, as witnessed by the strong female predominance in eating disorders (Hudson et al., 2007). The tendency of substance use disorders to be more frequent in males, although consistent (Office of Applied Studies, 2004), is open to several explanations. Perhaps men drown their sorrows in drink rather than get depressed. Thus there could be a common endophenotype for mood and substance use disorders, expressed differently in different genders (Winokur, 1979). But it is also possible that men carry a genetic risk for substance use that women do not. Finally, cultural factors affect prevalence, such as the tendency of men to bond with each other through drinking.

Personality disorders also show gender differences. Antisocial personality disorder (ASPD) is more common in men (Coid et al., 2007; Lenzenweger et al., 2007). Criminality, one of the main features of this diagnosis, is much more frequent in males (Hagan, 2008). Borderline personality disorder (BPD) is a mirror-image of ASPD, in that most clinical cases are female (Zimmerman et al., 2005). However, epidemiological studies in the United States (Lenzenweger et al., 2007) and in the United Kingdom (Coid et al., 2006) have found that BPD (contrary to ASPD) affects as many men as women in the community. The difference in clinical populations reflects help-seeking behavior and the fact that women with BPD are more likely to show suicidality than criminality, and it is possible that these disorders might share an endophenotype

(Paris, 1997). And most of the completed suicides in young people found on psychological autopsy to have a diagnosis of BPD occur in males (Lesage et al., 1994; McGirr et al., 2007), consistent with the overall higher rate of suicide in men.

Differences between males and females in eating disorders can be largely attributed to cultural forces. Women in modern societies are much more concerned about remaining thin than are men, a preoccupation that emerges only in societies where food is abundant (Garner & Garfinkel, 1980). In general, attractiveness in women is linked to physical attributes that suggest fertility, whereas in men attractiveness depends less on appearance and more on access to resources (Buss, 2007).

Some differences in prevalence might also be attributed to men being more aggressive than women; this is one of the most consistent findings in all gender research (Krahe, 2007). Men are clearly more physically aggressive and tend to do more harm to others than to themselves. But when they fail in life, men more likely than are women to kill themselves (Beautrais, 2001).

In summary, gender differences in mental disorders are real. They should not be regarded as social constructs or as attempts to marginalize one gender or another. Such differences do not in any way undermine the validity of mental disorders or affect their classification in DSM-5.

Culture: The prevalence of mental disorders is greatly affected by culture, by history, and by social context (Gone & Kirmayer, 2010). One does not to have to search far to see these relationships.

Culture shapes mental disorders in three ways. First, social forces influence how vulnerabilities to psychopathology (i.e., endophenotypes) express themselves in symptoms. Shorter (1994) has described a "symptom pool" in which distressed patients can show distress in different ways at different times that are shaped by culture. An example is that patients in the nineteenth century were more likely to present somatic complaints of various kinds ("classical hysteria"), whereas patients a hundred years later were more likely to come to treatment with psychological complaints such as anxiety and depression. Another example is the clinical presentation of eating disorders over the last few decades (Nasser et al., 2001). Although anorexia nervosa has been described in the medical literature for about 200 years, bulimia nervosa is a new syndrome that has now become common, largely through social contagion (Crandall, 1988). Thus bulimic patients express their distress through abnormal eating behavior, and the pattern has become a social epidemic.

The second way in which culture can shape mental disorders is by adding social stress to pre-existing biological vulnerabilities. This mechanism has been shown to apply to depression (Kendler, 2005) but may also apply to psychoses, long considered to be primarily biological disorders. Studies of immigrants have established that social disadvantage plays a role in its pathogenesis of schizophrenia (Dutta & Murray, 2010). The exact mechanism is not clear, but West Indian immigrants to the United Kingdom have a much higher rate of schizophrenia than those who remain in their native country, indicating that some form of social causation must be involved.

The third mechanism is that social forces can shape unique disorders that are only seen in one culture or a group of cultures—in which case the syndrome is described as "culture-bound" (Prince & Tseng-Laroche, 1990). Anorexia nervosa is unknown in societies where food is scarce (and where obesity is an advantage) and only develops in those where there is an excess of food (and in which obesity is a social disadvantage).

The question has sometimes been raised as to which mental disorders are universal. The answer is that by and large, the most severe conditions are seen in societies across the world, an observation that applies to schizophrenia (Jablensky et al., 1992), as well as bipolar disorder and melancholic depression (Weissman et al., 1996). However, precise prevalence can vary from one country to another, as well as between different ethnic groups within the same country. As noted, the rate of schizophrenia in immigrants is unusually high, much greater than in their countries of origin (Cantor-Graae & Selten, 2005).

In summary, culture plays an important role in the phenomenology and prognosis of mental disorder and is in some cases an etiological factor. DSM-5 recognizes these principles and includes a Cultural Formulation Interview consisting of 14 questions. We do not know much about the validity of this instrument or whether it is likely to be used in practice.

TREATMENT RESPONSE AS A SOURCE OF VALIDITY

Diagnosis can sometimes be validated by the application of a specific therapy. It is gratifying when the identification of a disease process leads logically to treatment. This scenario is most obvious in infectious diseases but also applies to a number of other diagnoses, from essential hypertension to cancer. Of course, some therapies, such as steroids or anti-inflammatory agents, have nonspecific effects on many disease processes. Yet even in conditions in which the etiology of certain illnesses is entirely unknown (e.g., cancer), treatment can be standardized.

The situation in psychiatry is more complex. Most diagnoses in the DSM manual cannot be used to prescribe definitive or consistent therapy. By and large, clinicians treat symptoms rather than disorders. Some therapies (e.g., antipsychotics and lithium) seem to target underlying neurobiological processes, even if we do not understand the mechanism. Many interventions control specific symptoms without reversing a disease process. Even in schizophrenia, drugs have more effects on positive than on negative symptoms, and although they can prevent relapses, have limited effects on the ultimate progression of the disorder. Similarly, lithium, although a great breakthrough, controls symptoms effectively but does not reverse the long-term course of bipolar disorder.

Frances and Egger (1999) summarized the strengths and limitations of DSM-IV in the light of research. Their conclusion was sobering: "We are at the epicycle stage of psychiatry where astronomy was before Copernicus and biology before Darwin." There seems no reason to change that assessment with the publication of DSM-5.

Chapter 5

Dimensionality

Science can describe phenomena using names or numbers. Categories are qualitative, while dimensions are quantitative. Some things in nature, such as the periodic table of elements, neatly fit a categorical paradigm. Others either have fuzzy edges or do not fit into categories at all. This problem has led to debates about the number of planets in the solar system, the hierarchical classification of biological species, the difference between life and non-life, and the nature of subatomic particles. Most of these disputes depend on where to draw a line to define a category. Many things are better described on a continuum.

Yet cognitive science consistently shows that people prefer to think in categories (Rosch & Lloyd, 1978). Medicine has always classified illness in that way. When experienced physicians assess a new patient, they do not go through an extensive checklist of signs and symptoms to make a diagnosis. Rather, they take one look at a patient, ask a few key questions, rapidly develop a hypothesis, and test it through further history-taking and examination procedures (Groopman, 2007). Thus categorical diagnoses correspond closely to what happens in a clinical encounter. Categories describe typicality in a clinical picture, are the basis of differential diagnosis, are practical for communication, and help determine treatment planning.

DSM-5 accepts categories provisionally but views them as artificial, proposing scoring procedures, wherever possible, to turn names into numbers. These scores are described as "dimensions," a geometrical metaphor that reflects a quantitative approach to psychopathology. The uncertainty of psychiatric diagnosis certainly supports a suspicion of categorical diagnoses, given that most categories in DSM consist of a set of symptoms that may or may not correspond to a coherent pathological entity. Thus even when diagnoses are useful guideposts, they do not correspond to Platonic reality. Moreover, categories become reified with time (Hyman, 2010) and are seen as if they were just as real as medical conditions with known biological markers.

Major depression is a prominent example—a set of symptoms that may or may not correspond to a coherent diagnostic entity associated with a unique endophenotype. Yet despite teaching psychiatry for many years, I have been unable to convince my students that making this diagnosis does not provide specific guidance for clinical management. For most trainees, major depression closes the case for writing a prescription.

Major depression fades imperceptibly into the sadness that everyone feels from time to time (Horwitz & Wakefield, 2007). Using a cut-off, as in DSM's category of major depression, 5 of 9 criteria (as opposed to say, 7 or 8 of 9) is an arbitrary procedure. That is why this category is so heterogeneous. Of course, patients with subclinical symptoms (less than 5) still suffer distress. It is also not clear that patients who have more than five criteria are fundamentally different from those who only barely meet the cut-off. The number 5, chosen because it is more than half of 9, is not scientific. Different levels of severity, or even separate disease processes, are obscured by a single category. Despite its ubiquity, major depression is one of the most problematic diagnoses in psychiatry.

Categorical classification imposes an artificial order when boundaries between disorders (or between disorders and normality) are fuzzy. Diagnostic categories are always *dichotomous*, allowing only for a yes or no decision. Those who do not quite meet criteria will be excluded, and patients with different levels of severity can get the same diagnosis. This process leads to a loss of information (Krueger et al., 2011).

Categories are the basis of differential diagnosis, but that procedure only makes sense when disease mechanisms are known. When they are not understood, as is almost always the case in psychiatry, differential diagnosis is guesswork. It should be kept in mind that the most important illness categories in current use, including well-researched diagnoses such as schizophrenia, may or may not meet the test of time.

The problems of diagnostic categories in psychiatry are many, including an inadequate scientific base, excessive comorbidity, inadequate coverage, an arbitrary boundary with normality, and heterogeneity among persons sharing the same diagnosis (Kraemer et al., 2004). Comorbidity, when massive, is a good sign that a category is not valid. Inadequate coverage is reflected by the fact many patients do not fit into the categories listed in the system. The "not otherwise specified" (NOS) option introduced in DSM-III has been used as a "wastebasket" for patients who do not meet criteria for any specific diagnosis within a group of disorders. In personality disorders, as many as 50% of cases only fit into an NOS category (Zimmerman et al., 2005). Moreover, the entire DSM system suffers from an artificial boundary between pathology and normality. Finally, categories obscure clinically important differences between patients meeting criteria for the same diagnosis. These are serious problems requiring a serious solution.

An overlap between categories leads patients to meet criteria for multiple diagnoses. This "comorbidity" reflects the absence of hierarchical rules: the DSM-IV-TR system did not generally allow clinicians to determine whether one diagnosis is primary and one secondary. Multiple diagnoses are actually a marker for severity; a community survey in the United Kingdom (Weich et al., 2011) found that those who meet criteria for several mental disorders have more severe levels of dysfunction.

The problem with comorbidity is that we have no definite way to determine whether one of two overlapping categories (e.g., mood disorder vs. anxiety disorder, or conduct disorder vs. attention deficit disorder) should take precedence over the other. If you follow the rules, you are *forced* to make more than one diagnosis. Comorbidity would be greatly reduced if DSM rewrote diagnostic criteria to minimize overlap. But lacking a clear justification, previous editions of the manual have been reluctant to do this. The problem could in principle be made irrelevant by replacing categories with dimensions.

A second problem is how to establish a boundary between pathology and normality. Many clinical symptoms blend into subclinical phenomena that can be seen in large sections of community populations. In other words, most people have periods when they are moody, unhappy, nervous, or show features of addiction. Many have suffered from *some* of the symptoms of common mental disorders. Even hallucinations can occur in normal people (Stip & Letourneau, 2009). Again, there is no definite cut-off point at which mental disorder can be said to be present.

A third issue is that neo-Kraepelinian categories in psychiatry rarely have robust relationships to biological measures, such as genetic markers, hormonal variations, or neuroimaging. By and large, relationships are stronger with dimensional scales that measure traits or score signs and symptoms (Kupfer & Regier, 2011). The problem is that diagnostic categories are *dichotomous*, allowing only for a yes-or-no decision. Those who do not quite meet criteria will be excluded, and patients with different levels of severity can receive the same diagnosis.

In summary, psychiatric diagnosis has an inadequate scientific base, including massive comorbidity, inadequate coverage leading many patients to fit only into a NOS option, while categories obscure clinically important differences between patients meeting criteria for the same diagnosis (Kraemer et al., 2004). These difficulties have led to the conclusion that categorical diagnosis in psychiatry should either be scrapped or kept only as a short-term expedient (Kupfer & Regier, 2011). Thus diagnosis would gradually become *dimensional*: rather than slotting patients into rigid categories, they would receive a score on one or more dimensions of psychopathology. Categorical overlap would eventually disappear. Patients would be given multiple scores rather than being packaged within a single category. All mental disorders would be seen as lying on one or several spectra reflecting neurobiological variability (Insel et al., 2010).

This is the basis of the "research domain criteria" (RDoCs) proposed by the National Institute of Mental Health (Insel et al., 2010). This model reflects the same point of view as DSM-5. But dimensionality denies any absolute boundary between disorder and normality. It offers the promise of a more scientific system but makes assumptions that may or may not correspond to empirical reality.

WHAT DO DIMENSIONS MEASURE?

Despite all their virtues, dimensions cannot untie the Gordian knot of validity for diagnostic classification in psychiatry. The reason is that dimensions suffer from most of the same limitations that afflict categorical systems. They are not based on a fundamental understanding of the etiology and pathogenesis of mental disorders. They are just as based on clinical observation as any categorical diagnosis. Until we know more about psychopathology, such a system can be no further advanced than medical diagnosis was in the nineteenth century, prior to the development of blood tests and X-rays. Diagnosis must be rooted in independent markers, most of which have to be biological. That would be true construct validity. At this point psychiatry can only aspire to having such measures. Converting clinical observations into dimensional scores will not solve the problem.

Dimensions may do a better job of measuring severity. It has been consistently shown that effects on functioning provide a better predictor of prognosis than categorization (Krueger & Bezdjian, 2009). However, the scoring of severity in psychiatry is not like the staging of tumors, based on imaging and pathological findings. Rather, the procedure is entirely rooted in observation and/or self-report data. If severity ratings are little but a count of signs and symptoms, then their introduction could be premature (First, 2005). In short, observable phenomena provide only indirect clues to underlying endophenotypes—the pathological processes that lie behind signs and symptoms. Until psychiatry understands mental illness better, the use of dimensions can only be a rough-and-ready expedient.

DIMENSIONS AND CLINICAL UTILITY

A system designed for practitioners as well as researchers has to have clinical utility. If dimensional diagnosis ends up not being used, for lack of clinical utility, adopting it would be pointless (First, 2010). Although taking blood pressure is simple, that is an objective physical measurement using a standard machine. Physicians learn how to perform complex diagnostic procedures (e.g., electrocardiograms) that can make useful predictions about the nature and course of disease. But there is no equivalent procedure in psychiatry.

The scoring of symptoms by practitioners, recommended in DSM-5, has limited utility. Clinicians would need a fair amount of training to rate symptoms in a valid way. Busy practitioners are likely to produce unreliable ratings. This procedure is also different from administering self-report questionnaires, which have been developed over years to establish their psychometric properties and that are the basis of most dimensional research in psychopathology. Such scales do not require reliable rating and are backed up by systematic testing. Research psychologists like these measures—they are accustomed to dealing with data in this way, and have long developed assessment instruments that use dimensional approaches. But it is usually impractical to ask patients to fill out questionnaires, even in a waiting room. And even when they do, the answers they give may not correspond to what clinicians observe.

Crucially, although dimensions give an impression of being more "scientific," they have not been shown to be valid in relation to etiology, pathogenesis, outcome, or choice of treatment. Scores based on symptoms cannot measure the underlying processes behind psychopathology. At this point, that idea has to be taken on faith. Until more data come in, it seems futile to ask clinicians (who already find DSM-IV to be burdensome) to learn an even more complex system. Most will find dimensional scoring unwieldy.

One reason is that the scoring of symptoms by practitioners requires using a Likert scale that clinicians need to be *trained* to use. But resistance on the part of clinicians to using dimensional scales is not based on habit or laziness (First, 2005). They know that scoring actually tells them no more than what they can readily observe. Why go through a complex procedure when an experienced clinician can know what is wrong in the first 5 minutes?

At present only a few dimensional measures have been used widely. Although scoring systems have been recommended for personality disorders (Costa & Widiger, 2001), for psychoses (Rosenman et al., 2003), and for depression (Korszun et al., 2004), none of the existing scales has a clinical following. No one is convinced that scoring tells you more about outcome and treatment than a categorical diagnosis.

I have emphasized that dimensional diagnosis tends to deny the existence of a separation between pathology and normality. Although disorder can sometimes be a matter of degree, if one were to follow dimensionality to its logical conclusion, *everyone* would merit a score reflecting some level of active or potential condition. Physicians in general medicine do sometimes think in this way, as shown by the widespread measurement of blood lipids in asymptomatic patients. But one need not confuse risk factors with disease. Unless we want to give up diagnosis entirely, we still need to establish cut-off points to distinguish true cases of mental disorder from subclinical or normal variants. Medicine is the study of disease, not a description of normal variation.

DIMENSIONS AND RESEARCH

A former director of the National Institute of Mental Health (Hyman, 2011) notes that when he was in charge, millions of dollars were spent on genetic studies of DSM categories, but the money was almost entirely wasted. The reason was that psychiatric diagnoses are not true endophenotypes (Regier et al., 2009); dimensionalization is more in accord with modern genetics (Hyman, 2010). Hyman is right about the danger of reifying categories, but dimensions also lack strong empirical support. Nonetheless, the current leaders of NIMH have suggested directing funding away from existing DSM categories to a future "brain-based" system (RDoCS; Insel, 2009; Insel et al., 2010; Sanislow et al., 2010), which could be more closely related to endophenotypes, genes, and neural circuits than traditional categories. This is an interesting proposal that should be researched systematically. But at this point RDoCS is an idea that may or may not work out.

The principle that mental disorders are brain disorders has become a mantra. It is not a fact but an ideology used to validate psychiatry as a discipline. It represents that hope that mental illness can be translated into neuroscience. It has even been suggested that psychiatry should reunite with neurology into one specialty that treats brain diseases (Insel & Quirion, 2002). (A neurological colleague once quipped, "We treat the axon and you treat the synapse.")

I do not agree that psychiatry can be reduced to the clinical application of neuroscience. Needless to say, neuroscience is a valuable tool for our specialty. But studying mental processes on their own terms is an equally valid strategy. Mind is an *emergent* property of the brain and cannot be fully explained on a cellular or molecular level. In other words, complex systems yield phenomena that "emerge" from simpler components but are not fully determined by them. In the simplest example, the properties of water are not explained by the atomic structure of hydrogen or oxygen. Although reducing a system to its components sheds light on what can be directly observed, explanations of mental disorder should eventually be based on several different levels of analysis, from genes and neurons to psychosocial processes.

Thus, the holy grail of neuroscience may never provide a complete resolution of the problems raised by diagnostic classification. Research in recent decades has taught us much about the brain. Imaging studies have identified specific functions for many cortical and subcortical structures. We have learned about the alarm system in the amygdala, the memory system in the hippocampus, the reward system in the nucleus accumbens, and the behavioral control system in the prefrontal cortex. At the same time, biochemical and physiological studies have defined synaptic pathways by which neurons communicate, as well as cellular pathways by which proteins are constructed and used within a neuron. Research could eventually specify the genes and proteins that shape all these processes.

One can only applaud these scientific advances. However, none of this research has thus far had *any* clinical application—either to the understanding of disease mechanisms or to the treatment of mental illness. Molecular genetics and neuroimaging have not explained why people become psychotic or severely depressed. It remains possible that future editions of DSM will be guided by helpful neurobiological markers—but not this time around.

The gap between basic and clinical science is no accident. Mental processes are too complex to be readily reduced to neuroscience. Moreover, brain mechanisms are only one of several relevant levels of analysis, and a comprehensive theory also needs to include psychological and social mechanisms. Biological reductionism in psychiatry supports a practice based almost entirely on drug treatment. In a widely cited article by Insel and Quirion (2002), the word "psychological" does not even appear. This mindless approach to psychiatry has consequences for practice.

SCORING SYMPTOMS

One way to dimensionalize mental disorders is to score the number of symptoms present in a patient. Thus, if there are nine criteria for a diagnosis, and each is rated simply "yes," "maybe," or "no," then one would immediately have a scale ranging from 0 to 27. Alternatively, clinicians could score each criterion on a 4-point "Likert scale" (not at all, some, a fair amount, or a lot). In principle, the procedure could be applied to any diagnosis. However severity scores would not produce dimensions in the same way as scores on a test. There is no way of knowing how to weigh each criterion. Psychometric analysis of questionnaires requires that a large number of items be analyzed to ensure that the instrument as a whole produces a reliable result. Likert scales have to be smoothly continuous, not bumpy. Reaching that goal usually requires years of research.

Scoring existing diagnostic criteria creates a chimerical beast that is neither fully categorical nor properly dimensional. Although the criteria in the manual can be useful in the aggregate, hardly any of them has been shown to have validity on their own. Many reflect symptoms that resemble each other and often occur together. This is why even sophisticated statistical methods (such as factor analysis) cannot "carve nature at its joints." Ideally, a valid dimensional scale would need to be created de novo and, based on sources of external validity, not on existing criteria. DSM-5 does not have the evidence to support such a procedure nor the time to develop it. That is why scoring of severity was moved to the Appendix.

DIAGNOSTIC SPECTRA

Overlapping diagnoses that reflect different aspects of the same pathological process may fall within *spectra*, a range of disorders rooted in common mechanisms. The oldest and best supported is the schizophrenia spectrum (Siever & Davis, 1991). This concept includes conditions ranging from severe psychosis (schizophrenia itself and milder psychoses (brief psychotic episodes and delusional disorder) to diagnoses in which formal delusions and hallucinations are absent (schizotypal personality disorder). The validity of this concept is supported by family studies, in which spectrum disorders show a stronger pattern of inheritance than does schizophrenia alone (Kendler et al., 1994). It has also long been known that schizotypal personality shares biological markers with overt schizophrenia, even if they are not specific enough to be used for diagnosis (Siever, 2007).

The concept of a mood spectrum also has a degree of validity. Several decades ago, the American psychiatrist George Winokur suggested that depression and alcoholism might reflect the same disease process—with the former being more common in women and the latter being more common in men (Winokur et al., 1975). Later, the Swiss psychiatrist Jules Angst proposed a more restricted spectrum, including classical depression and its subclinical variants, as well as conditions sharing the same endophenotype, particularly anxiety disorders (Angst & Merikangas, 1997).

Other spectra have been proposed for panic/agoraphobia, substance use, psychosis as a whole, anorexia-bulimia, an obsessive-compulsive domain, and social anxiety (Frank et al., 2011). A bipolar spectrum (to be discussed in Chapter 8) would bring together all disorders in psychiatry in which mood instability is prominent (Ghaemi et al., 2002). Another concept is an impulsive spectrum (Zanarini, 1993), based on evidence that impulsive traits (present in substance abuse, eating disorders, and personality disorders), run in the same families.

Spectra could be used to search for endophenotypes (biological pathways) that lie behind symptoms (Gottesman & Gould, 2003). But like dimensions, they all still depend on phenomenological observation. In the absence of biological markers, disorders may not fall within the same spectrum just because they resemble each other. And disorders may also be based on multiple endophenotypes, in which case basing spectra on clinical features alone would oversimplify a complex problem.

How many diagnostic spectra would we need to describe most of the disorders listed in the DSM manual? An earlier study using factor analysis (Krueger, 1999) suggested that most of the territory could be covered by two factors: internalizing and externalizing disorders. However, these dimensions do not describe cognitive impairment, a central issue for psychiatry. More recently, Kotov et al. (2011) suggested that five dimensions would do the trick: internalizing, externalizing, cognitive, somatoform, and antagonism. Thus, *internalizing* dimensions would describe most anxiety and mood disorders; *externalizing* would describe substance use and impulsive disorders; *cognitive* would describe schizophrenia, neurodevelopmental disorders, and neurocognitive disorders; *somatoform* would describe somatic symptom disorders; and *antagonism* would account for personality disorders. There may be something useful to be garnered from these factor analyses. But keep in mind that they only describe symptomatic resemblances and tell you nothing about etiology or pathogenesis.

A SCALE FOR SUICIDE ASSESSMENT

DSM-5 offers one dimensional measure that has nothing to do with diagnosis at all. The manual takes a leap into clinical assessment and goes beyond the manual's mandate, proposing a scale for predicting suicide.

Every clinician is trained to assess suicide risk, using a melange of indicators such as stated intent, past suicidal behavior, psychosocial status, presence of substance abuse, family history, and clinical diagnosis (Bongar, 1992). Yet the clinical prediction of suicide has mostly been marked by failure (Paris, 2006). Empirical studies show, at best, a small relationship between predictors and outcome. Large-scale research using algorithms based on commonly applied clinical judgment fail to predict a single case (Goldstein et al., 1991). The sober fact is that psychiatrists are unable to determine which patients are at risk for taking their own lives. If they could, they might be in a position to prevent that outcome.

Why is this so? The reason is that although suicidal ideation is very common and although attempts are not infrequent, completed suicide is relatively rare. Because of this "base rate" problem, most methods of predicting suicide turn up an enormous number of false–positives. Even the most successful predictors, such as the Suicide Intent Scale (Beck et al., 1974), can only predict completion with statistical significance (Suominen et al., 2004). Even if one sees relationships in large samples, a scale can be wrong most of the time when applied in practice. Scores based on statistical data are usually not accurate enough to be useful in making clinical decisions. Although long-term follow-up studies have found that scales can have *some* predictive value, most people who score high on them never commit suicide (Goldstein et al., 1991). Thus, in the vast majority of cases, completion is not predictable in practice.

The failure of prediction has an important corollary. Most people who are admitted to hospital as suicide risks are unlikely to kill themselves (Paris, 2006). And those who carry the greatest risk may never present clinically. The vast majority of completed suicides occur on the very first attempt and involve guns or hanging (Beautrais, 2001).

DSM-5, responding understandably to clinical need, but with a weak scientific basis, has jumped into the breech. Although its scale assesses some standard risk factors (previous attempt, aggressivity, social isolation, recent losses, chronic pain, diagnosis of severe mental disorder, substance abuse, suicidal plans, and hopelessness), it only has face validity, mirroring what psychiatrists have long been taught about the assessment of suicide risk but not providing scientific justification for clinical prediction. Like much else in DSM-5, this scale offers only an illusion of scientific validity. It has not been validated and does not belong in a diagnostic manual. Perhaps it was too much to expect for psychiatrists to admit they cannot predict who will and who will not commit suicide. But scales like this need to be well validated. It will be one of the most unscientific sections of DSM-5. But given the need of clinicians to *feel* they can make such predictions, it could be widely used.

DIMENSIONALIZATION AS A VISION

The American journalist Lincoln Steffens, who visited the Soviet Union shortly after the Russian Revolution, famously concluded, "I have been over into the future, and it works." It took decades for everyone to realize just how wrong he was.

Similarly, the editors of DSM-5 have a visionary view of psychiatric diagnosis. They know where psychiatry is going and want to help it get there more rapidly. Dimensionalization is a major factor in their ideology. But only time will tell whether it works for or against clinical practice.

First nicely summarizes the issues:

"For there to be any chance that the DSM-5 dimensions will fare better than their DSM-IV predecessors, significant efforts must be made to establish their reliability, sensitivity to change, and clinical utility. Fundamental to this effort is empirical evidence establishing not only that clinicians find such measures "feasible" or "acceptable," but also that the use of such measures improve clinical outcomes. Otherwise it is unlikely that clinicians will be motivated to spend the time and effort required to put the measures into routine clinical use." (2010, p. 698)

The situation would be different if dimensions had the scientific status of physical measurements such as blood pressure. As it stands, the only practical issue for practitioners is whether a disorder is mild, moderate, or severe. But severity does not define the boundaries of disorders, and there is also no established benefit to a scoring system that simply counts criteria. Clinicians who want to communicate about their patients can do just as well by continuing to use categories. And that this is exactly what they will do.

Chapter 6

Clinical Utility

DSM-5 needs to be practical. Busy practitioners will not use a diagnostic classification in the same way as researchers. The success of the new edition will stand or fall on whether clinicians apply it in daily practice.

Practitioners like familiar diagnoses. Whatever problems there are with the boundaries of mental disorders, typical cases of well-established categories, such as schizophrenia or bipolar illness, immediately convey a great deal of information. Every psychiatry and psychology student learns about these diagnoses and knows, more or less, what a case looks like. That is why some prefer prototypes, even if diagnosis over the last 30 years has made them comfortable with algorithms.

Eventually research may provide us with sufficient reasons to abandon familiar categories. Major depression, conduct disorder, and schizophrenia could turn out to be a group of disorders rather than one. When the evidence is strong enough, we can replace the old with the new. But until we have that kind of data, traditional concepts remain valuable. DSM-5 is too keen to be innovative, even when data are not yet in.

Making it more difficult to reach a diagnosis undermines recognition of disorders. If a system is too complicated to use, practitioners will not reach accurate conclusions. Therefore, a lack of clinical utility is bad for patients, who may end up receiving useless or harmful treatment. All the potential advantages of creating a new edition of DSM could be lost.

Consider an example of how clinicians use manuals in the real world: the familiar category of major depressive disorder. Research shows that only a minority follow DSM rules in making this diagnosis (Zimmerman & Galione, 2010). Rather, they depend on a global impression or "prototype" and may not quite remember what the manual says. Few take the time to count to determine whether five of nine criteria are met. Psychologists have long known that the most anyone can remember from a list of any kind is seven items (which is why we have to write down telephone numbers). So who can remember nine criteria? You could use an acronym of capital letters to jog your memory. But you would still have to remember the acronym.

Because clinicians do not have the time to go through algorithimic procedures, they reach conclusions based on immediate impressions. This is what Kahneman (2011) has called "thinking fast." The problem with impressionistic diagnosis is that it is particularly prone to cognitive error, such as coming up with the first diagnosis that comes to mind (which Kahneman describes as an "availability heuristic").

All editions of DSM have clearly stated that they are not intended to be guides to treatment. But that is not what happens in practice. Clinicians go directly from diagnosis to treatment. Moreover, they prefer diagnoses that lead to a specific treatment of some kind, even when they are wrong. For example, patients who *say* they are depressed and have some accompanying symptoms, such as insomnia and fatigue, tend to be diagnosed with major depression, followed by a routine drug prescription. The overdiagnosis of major depression, based on its overly broad definition, is one of the most serious problems in contemporary psychiatry. Although some patients meeting these criteria benefit from antidepressants, results are far from consistent, as shown by placebo-controlled trials (Kirsch et al., 2008) and by effectiveness research (Valenstein, 2006).

Most categories in DSM-5 are syndromes, not diseases. Because DSM criteria are little more than lists of symptoms, clinicians who use the manual end up treating symptoms rather than diseases. It is only the reification of diagnosis that gives the impression that a category such as "major depression" is a specific medical illness that responds to specific methods of treatment.

DIAGNOSIS AS COMMUNICATION

The most important function of diagnosis is *communication*—to other practitioners, to patients, to families, and to health-care system administrators (First et al., 2004). Yet if clinicians find DSM-5 categories unwieldy, they will not be used effectively.

Diagnosis also provides important information for people suffering from mental disorders. There was a time when psychiatrists were reluctant to share diagnoses with patients. I was taught to practice that way. It was also a time when physicians were much more authoritarian than they are now, and the idea of educating patients to participate in their own treatment had not been developed. Moreover, because the diagnostic system used when I was in training (DSM-II) was flawed, we didn't think patients were missing much.

Some of my teachers believed that communicating a diagnosis could actually interfere with treatment, by pigeonholing patients into categories that failed to acknowledge unique life stories. My supervisors told me that the best answer to the question "What's my diagnosis, doctor?" should be "I don't think about your problems in that way." That answer was not quite honest, but my teachers, sympathetic to psychoanalysis, were afraid that diagnosis could become the *only* way to understand a patient. (Although they were wrong about so many other things, they were right to point out this danger.)

Like most psychiatrists, I gradually changed my ways. For the first time in the history of psychiatry, diagnosis made a real difference in the choice of treatment. The best example is bipolar disorder. In the early 1970s, with the introduction of lithium, it became crucially important to distinguish bipolarity from schizophrenia. One also needed to educate bipolar patients about their disorder to help them to be compliant with treatment. Although some did not want to hear about their diagnosis (particularly when in a manic mood), psychoeducation can be useful when bipolar patients are euthymic (Scott et al., 2006).

Each diagnosis in psychiatry presents unique challenges for patient education. Schizophrenia, which interferes with insight, presents particular difficulties. I often tried to explain this diagnosis to patients, with very limited success. Only in recent years have formal cognitive therapy programs been developed to make use of more sophisticated psychoeducational methods (Rummel-Kluge & Kissling, 2008).

It is now widely accepted that treatment benefits from informing patients about their diagnosis. I am familiar with its use in my own area of subspecialization, borderline personality disorder (BPD). This is a disabling condition marked by unstable mood, impulsivity, and unstable relationships (Paris, 2008b). In pioneer research on the management of these patients, Linehan (1993) described how the first step of her treatment method (dialectical behavior therapy) was to show a slide of the DSM criteria, explain the diagnosis in detail, and use the criteria as guideposts for planning treatment. My experience confirms the value of these procedures. I have found that explaining the diagnosis brings most patients relief, as they realize that their problems are known to psychiatry and that research on treatment can guide their recovery. I encourage patients to look up the diagnosis and to discuss with me which features they have and which ones they don't.

In modern medical practice, patients are no longer passive consumers of services. Many read about their illness on the Internet. Some arrive in the office armed with printouts. Patients need to know—and deserve to know—their diagnosis. Moreover, each major disorder now has support groups devoted to explaining the nature of the problem to patients and to their families. All these developments make it even more important that DSM-5 diagnoses be user-friendly. However, it is not clear how easily clinicians can explain complex diagnoses, particularly if they are based on scoring procedures.

MAKING DIAGNOSIS USER-FRIENDLY

DSM-III demanded more of clinicians than did its predecessors. Because the manual was extremely popular and came to dominate the mental health field, everyone was expected to use it. Moreover, clinicians became familiar with its specific criteria, even if few went through the procedure of counting them. Academics and researchers went a step further, using structured interviews that were much more reliable than clinical diagnosis (i.e., based on DSM criteria, but forcing clinicians to go through an algorithm thoroughly and systematically).

There was little formal research about how previous editions of DSM were actually used. Jampala et al. (1992) surveyed psychiatric educators and residents, with results (unsurprisingly) showing that the manuals were consulted by almost everyone. For example, psychiatric social workers routinely make DSM diagnoses, largely because insurance companies require them to do so (Frazer et al., 2009). What these surveys fail to show is how diagnostic decisions are reached or whether the specific procedures required in the manual were followed.

My experience, in line with the findings of Zimmerman and Galione (2010), has been that only a few clinicians are systematic and make algorithmic diagnoses in the way described by the manual. They have a general picture in their minds of what constitutes a major depression, a manic episode, or a panic attack and make a diagnosis if the patient's symptoms approximate that picture. Thus many clinicians still prefer to diagnose by *prototype*.

DSM may have expected too much of its users by asking them to follow algorithms. Clinicians are pressed for time and need to cut corners. They read the manual while in training and rarely consult it later. In discussing diagnostic dilemmas with colleagues, I almost never hear how many criteria for a disorder a patient met or what, precisely, were the observations on which each criterion was scored. I am much more likely to hear about one particular symptom believed to be characteristic of a diagnosis.

THE DEMISE OF THE FIVE-AXIS SYSTEM

The five-Axis system introduced by DSM-III was noble in theory but unworkable in practice. Its concept, providing multiple perspectives on diagnosis, was well intentioned. Who could argue with the need to identify personality traits and disorders on Axis II, with the scoring of medical conditions on Axis III, stressors on Axis IV, and functioning on Axis V? But clinicians focused on Axis I—the traditional way of making categorical diagnoses. Most reports stopped there. Axis II (personality disorders and intellectual disability) was a second-class citizen, mostly ignored or at best "deferred." Axis III (medical diagnoses) was not always of interest, and Axis IV (stressors) had a vague rating that was difficult to score. Axis V was a problematic amalgam of symptoms and psychosocial functioning. For all these reasons, the five-Axis system will not be missed. (One can only wonder whether the same judgment will be made about some of the innovations of DSM-5 when DSM-6 is ready for publication.)

Yet although diagnosis is a meaningful cluster of symptoms, it does not always reflect functioning. We need a separate measure for that. Some people with serious mental disorders manage surprisingly well, whereas some patients with mild to moderate mental disorders function at a low level. Even in schizophrenia, 10% to 20% of patients are employed, depending on the job market (Marwaha & Johnson, 2004). Nearly one-fourth of men with schizophrenia (and about half of women) will eventually marry and have families (Saugstad, 1989). At the same time, patients with common mental disorders (anxiety and depression) can be unemployed and socially isolated.

Axis V was a failure because it mixed apples and oranges. It tried to account for symptom severity, ability to work, and the quality of intimate relationships—all in one number! The results were predictably unreliable and misleading. In some ways, the failure of Axis V was instructive. Introduced in DSM-III, it was based on a measure developed years before by Luborsky (1962), the Health-Sickness Rating Scale (HSRS), and later adapted into a Global Assessment Scale (GAS; Endicott et al., 1976). The GAS was renamed in DSM-III-R as the Global Assessment of Functioning (GAF). The concept was to score functioning on a scale from 0 to 100. In case of a discrepancy between different areas of functioning (as one often sees), the score should reflect the lowest common denominator, so that the most dysfunctional area would determine the final score. DSM-III also asked clinicians, as a way of assessing change, to record a score for the highest level in the past year, which could then be compared to the current GAF.

For the last 30 years, I have taught residents to write clinical reports that include a GAF score. They almost never get it right. The reason is that the number is a composite. A patient could be unemployed and isolated but only have mild symptoms. Or they could have severe symptoms despite having a good job and a loving family. All could receive the same GAF score. In practice, the GAF functions not as a 100-point but a 30-point scale. Any score higher than 80 would be Utopia, and I don't think I have ever felt that good for a week. Patients who score between

70 and 80 are having expectable reactions to situations, which define them as mentally healthy. We don't see patients like that. People with mental disorders always score below 70. Thus a patient with only mild dysfunction would fall between 60 and 70, moderate problems between 50 and 60, and severe dysfunction below 50. This leaves a very narrow range. Finally, the GAF scale lacked clinical utility. Almost none of my colleagues (including most of those who used to be my students) could follow its complex procedures.

DSM-5 eliminated Axis V but did not come up with anything better. A system called Patient-Reported Outcomes Measurement Information System (PROMIS; Anatchkova & Bjorner, 2010) could be used both as a measure of functioning and of disability (Narrow et al., 2009; Narrow & Kuhl, 2011). But its scientific basis is uncertain, and it is much more complicated than GAF, virtually guaranteeing that it will never be used in clinical practice. In the end, DSM decided to recommend that to rate disability, the World Health Organization Disability Assessment Schedule (*www.who.int/entity/classifications/icf/whodasii/en/index.html*) can be used.

The clinical utility of this option remains in doubt. In the 30-plus years that I taught DSM-III and DSM-IV to residents, I was unable to get them to use the five-Axis system with accuracy. Multiple scoring is cumbersome and burdensome. If the new system requires many minutes of thought, then the task will almost certainly be left undone. You can only ask clinicians to make that kind of effort if doing so has real clinical value. Busy practitioners will not take the time to do complex scoring when they can directly observe symptoms. They will rebel at completing 5-point scales, however beloved these procedures are for some research psychologists. That procedure would only be worthwhile if it could provide a practical link to treatment—as in oncology, where staging of cancers has a real use in planning therapy.

Once, when I challenged a colleague on one of the work groups about the complexity of some of the DSM-5 criteria, he replied, "But physicians learn how to read electrocardiograms." Nice try, but this is a false analogy. There can be no comparison between the measurement of electrical waves and clinical observation.

Psychiatry is many decades away from developing a classification based on etiology and pathogenesis (Hyman, 2007; First, 2010). Unfortunately, that has not led to humility among experts, and the tone of the DSM-5 website is often one of undeserved self-congratulation. Clinicians have to use this system for years to come, but it is only based on observation. Rather than introducing quasi-scientific methods, we should accept that DSM-5 system is provisional and at least make it user-friendly. Meanwhile we need to be patient and wait until we know enough to come up with something better.

PART II

SPECIFIC DIAGNOSES

Chapter 7

Schizophrenia Spectrum and Other Psychoses

I have always taught my students that the DSM system makes the most sense for categorizing severe mental disorders but has problems in classifying milder ones. Psychoses, marked by dramatic symptoms and severe dysfunction, are much like medical illnesses. One might, therefore, expect them to present easier diagnostic challenges than common mental disorders. Yet uncertainty about boundaries also afflicts psychoses. The core problem, once again, is that diagnosis based on phenomenology alone can never be more than approximate.

DEFINING THE SCHIZOPHRENIA SPECTRUM

The overall definition of schizophrenia in DSM-5 has not greatly changed from previous manuals. A patient must have at least two characteristic symptoms for at least a month: delusions, hallucinations, disorganized speech, abnormal psychomotor activity, negative symptoms (including at least one from the first three), social/occupational dysfunction, and a 6-month duration of illness. Previous criteria giving particular weight to bizarre delusions or Schneiderian hallucinations have been removed, as there is no evidence these symptoms are pathognomonic. The traditional subtypes of schizophrenia have also been dropped. This was a good decision—although some of the older literature suggested that the paranoid type may be distinct, recent studies have not confirmed that conclusion (Tandon et al., 2008). Disorders assumed to lie in the schizophrenia spectrum are also listed: schizotypal personality disorder (also listed under personality disorders), schizophreniform disorder, brief psychotic disorder, and delusional disorder.

DIFFERENTIAL DIAGNOSIS OF SCHIZOPHRENIA AND BIPOLAR DISORDER

Kraepelin (1921) introduced a dichotomy between schizophrenia and bipolar disorder, based on course of illness. This idea has shaped psychiatry for almost a century. Kraepelin proposed that schizophrenia (then called "dementia praecox") is usually a chronic illness with a slow declining course, whereas bipolar disorder (then called "manic-depression") is usually an intermittent illness with periods of good functioning between episodes. (He acknowledged that some cases are difficult to put in one or the other category.) The Kraepelinian dichotomy became even more influential decades later, after the introduction of lithium, when differential diagnosis became of practical importance for choosing pharmacological treatment. But the distinction has been recently undermined by research findings.

Only some cases of bipolar disorder show remission between episodes, whereas others—particularly those with prominent psychotic symptoms—tend to develop severe and chronic psychosocial dysfunction (Goodwin & Jamison, 2007). Moreover, neither schizophrenia nor bipolar disorder "breed true"—patients in the same families can have one or the other condition (Craddock & Owen, 2005). Do these discrepancies reflect inaccuracy of diagnosis or a common diathesis for psychosis? The latter possibility is supported by twin studies showing an overlap in heritability (Cardno et al., 2002). A large-scale molecular genetic study found that patients with both diagnoses have similar alleles, suggesting that what is inherited could be a vulnerability to psychosis, rather than to a particular diagnosis (The International Schizophrenia Consortium, 2009).

Nonetheless, many experts have maintained that differences between these two conditions are real. The British psychiatrist Murray and his colleagues argued as follows:

> "…individuals with schizophrenia have more obvious brain structural and neuropsychological abnormalities than those

with bipolar disorder; and pre-schizophrenic children are characterized by cognitive and neuromotor impairments, which are not shared by children who later develop bipolar disorder. Furthermore, the risk-increasing effect of obstetric complications has been demonstrated for schizophrenia but not for bipolar disorder" (Murray et al., 2004, p. 405).

Lawrie et al. (2010) concluded:

"We acknowledge that there is overlap in genetic susceptibility, symptoms, treatments and prognoses between schizophrenia and bipolar disorder. Indeed, perhaps the most striking finding of recent genetic association and genome-wide association studies has been the degree of shared genetic susceptibility to schizophrenia and bipolar disorder. However, shared polygenic vulnerability does not necessarily imply that the resultant conditions lie on one continuum or even several continua. Indeed, there is considerable evidence for differences between the disorders in terms of risk factors, pathology and treatment response. Thus urban birth, abnormal neurodevelopment and premorbid cognitive impairment are strongly associated with schizophrenia but not with bipolar disorder. Schizophrenia is associated with an increased burden of large and rare chromosomal abnormalities (copy number variants) not seen in bipolar disorder. In addition there are replicated differences in brain structure and function between the disorders, which although primarily quantitative allow for considerable separation of the disorders. Most importantly, there are clearly established differences in responsiveness to lithium and other treatments."

These controversies might be resolved if schizophrenia and bipolar disorder were shown to be rooted in multiple, rather than single, diatheses. Thus, they could have genes in common and still be different diseases. In any case, genetic overlap reflects only one aspect of either illness, and other features could depend on different mechanisms.

At the beginning of the genomic era, it was hoped that molecular genetics would be a key to unlock psychoses and that specific disorders would be associated with a few specific alleles. These days, the consensus is that such a simple solution is unlikely. McClelland et al. (2007, p. 194) concluded that schizophrenia

> "....is highly heterogeneous genetically and that many predisposing mutations are highly penetrant and individually rare, even specific to single cases or families. This 'common disease— rare alleles' hypothesis is supported by recent findings in human genomics and by allelic and locus heterogeneity for other complex traits."

But genetic studies are not the only way to explore biological mechanisms. Although we all worship at the shrine of DNA, epigenetic mechanisms may be just as important. Finally, although biological markers could eventually be used for differential diagnosis (Benes, 2010), there is no sign that they are coming any time soon.

Differentiating schizophrenia and bipolar disorder would be an academic matter if it were not for the fact that diagnosis makes a real difference for choice of treatment. Both patient groups have responded to antipsychotics, but these drugs have more consistent preventive effects against recurrence in schizophrenia, whereas lithium is much more specific to bipolar disorder, both for acute treatment and for the prevention of relapse (Healy, 2009). In this respect, DSM-5 is right to maintain the distinction.

SCHIZOPHRENIA—ONE DISORDER OR MANY?

Schizophrenia may not be a disease but a syndrome. Its heterogeneity may be the reason why no biological markers have yet been found to be associated with the diagnosis. The classical subtypes used in DSM-IV (paranoid, disorganized, catatonic, undifferentiated, or residual) did not do a good job of dissecting schizophrenia, and all have been eliminated in DSM-5. These subcategories were taught to students for years, but research has never confirmed their validity (Linscott et al., 2009). In any case, subtypes were not commonly used in practice. Paranoid symptoms are associated with a later onset of disease, a less severe course, and fewer negative symptoms (Gottesman et al., 1982). But there is nothing specific about paranoid delusions, which can also be seen in mania, psychotic depression, delusional disorder, and dementia (Bentall et al., 2009). Catatonia, a term with a long history in psychiatry, may also not be specific to schizophrenia (Fink et al., 2009). In DSM-5, it is treated as a specifier rather than a subtype.

We do not understand why schizophrenia presents so differently in different patients. Why do some patients have striking negative symptoms, whereas others suffer from more florid positive symptoms? Kraepelinian concepts, now a hundred years old, lie on slippery ground. Renaming would also not solve the problem. Van Os (2009), concerned about as much about stigma as about validity, suggested the disorder be renamed as a "salience syndrome"—but this unfamiliar term is very unlikely to catch on. Few would be prepared to discard a concept so basic to psychiatry as schizophrenia, even if the name fails to describe the fundamental features of the illness. We will have to wait for a better understanding of the illness before we are in a position to give it a better name.

ATTENUATED PSYCHOSIS SYNDROME

One of the most controversial proposals for DSM-5 was the proposal for a category of risk psychosis—or, in its renamed version, *attenuated psychosis syndrome*. The diagnosis would be based on the presence of milder symptoms (but still including delusions, hallucinations, and disorganized speech) that are present at least once a week, progress over time, and cause disability, while leaving reality testing intact.

Early psychosis—that is, prodromal cases of schizophrenia—has been a major subject of research in recent years. Researchers have suggested that the treatment of first-episode psychosis might prevent sequelae (McGlashan & Johanessen, 1996; Addington et al., 2008), but the evidence is not there to support that idea. Research has not shown that early treatment in patients at risk actually prevents the development of the illness. A clinical trial of olanzapine failed to yield any benefits over placebo (McGlashan et al., 2006). A recent report (prominently highlighted in the media) has suggested that omega-3 fatty acids can slow or even prevent the onset of psychosis in high-risk groups (Amminger et al., 2010). But that is only one study—practice should not change until it is firmly replicated. Finally, cognitive therapy is also of no preventive value in these cases (Morrison et al., 2012). Thus, despite some promising recent research (Hegeland et al., 2012), we lack convincing evidence that early treatment of risk psychosis makes a difference in prognosis (McGorry et al., 2010).

It is difficult to give up hope of preventing such a serious illness. William Carpenter was the chair of the DSM-5 work group and is a senior schizophrenia researcher (he testified at the trial of John Hinckley in 1982). Citing data from a follow-up study of high-risk cases by Woods et al. (2009), Carpenter (2009) proposed that these patients could be identified, diagnosed, and successfully treated. In Australia, under the influence of prominent psychiatrist Patrick McGorry, a national program was put into place for early identification and treatment. But attenuated psychosis is not necessarily early psychosis.

Patients meeting the criteria for attenuated psychosis do have an increased risk for conversion to schizophrenia. The problem is the very large number of false–positives. One large-scale study (Cannon et al., 2008) found the conversion rate after 30 months was only 35%. That leaves two-thirds who would be treated unnecessarily. In practice, identification of attenuated psychosis could be become higher if, as shown by previous diagnostic epidemics, clinicians, who are trained not to "miss anything," are less cautious than researchers in identifying cases. Thus diagnosing people who are not ill would lead to treatment for those who will never develop schizophrenia, not to speak of stigmatization. This would be another example of DSM's "mission creep," in which a category spreads from clear-cut disease to near-normal problems. And once a diagnosis is accepted, it is almost certain that physicians will use it frequently, that concerned families will insist on treatment, and that a larger number of people will receive antipsychotic medication.

The problem with adding risk categories to a diagnostic manual is that nearly *everyone* is vulnerable to *some* form of mental illness. If we were to follow this precedent, then the entire population would almost certainly merit a psychiatric diagnosis. To justify making diagnoses in preclinical cases, one has to be sure that the risk is very high and/or make use of objective measures (as physicians do for pre-diabetes). In schizophrenia, we lack the science to predict who will go on to develop psychosis and who will not. That is why there is little basis for intervening in putative prodromal cases.

In May 2012, DSM chose *not* to adopt this diagnosis but relegated it to an Appendix containing conditions requiring further study. This was the right decision.

SOME UNRESOLVED PROBLEMS

The other categories of psychosis are more poorly understood than schizophrenia, and it is not even clear whether they belong in the same spectrum. The most clinically important example is delusional disorder, a condition one sees with some frequency in the clinic but about which research is thin. This poorly understood diagnosis is marked by delusions without thought disorder. It could be a form of schizophrenia or a unique form of psychopathology. A family study conducted in a community population (Kendler & Walsh, 2007) found delusional disorder related not to schizophrenia but to alcoholism. This surprising observation reminds us that these patients remain poorly understood. No changes in this category have been proposed for DSM-5. The definition describes delusions of at least 1-month duration that are not bizarre and that do not markedly impair functioning.

Another problem child is schizophreniform disorder, first introduced in DSM-III to account for cases that recover rapidly and do not progress to chronicity. The diagnosis is not often made, as briefer psychotic episodes resolve rapidly, whereas first-episode schizophrenic patients, who usually have a long duration of untreated psychosis, do not (McGlashan, 1999). In a family study, Kendler and Walsh (2007) found schizophreniform cases to be related to mood disorders, rather than to schizophrenia, supporting Kraepelin's concept of schizophrenia as a chronic disease. In DSM-5, clinicians are asked to rate whether good prognostic features are present, but we do not know whether doing so is clinically useful.

Finally, brief psychotic disorder (less than 1 month of symptoms, not accounted for by substance use) remains in DSM without revised criteria. It may or may not belong in the schizophrenia spectrum. There is little research on the outcome of such cases, so one cannot assume that they necessarily represent a first episode of schizophrenia.

FUTURE DIRECTIONS IN THE SCHIZOPHRENIA SPECTRUM

Schizophrenia remains a central concern for psychiatrists. We usually manage positive symptoms successfully, but negative symptoms tend to continue and have never been shown to be responsive to medication. The upside is that patients with schizophrenia usually get better in middle age, and most eventually stop coming to psychiatry (Harding et al., 1987).

The boundary problem in schizophrenia cannot currently be resolved because of a lack of biological markers to determine whether disease lies, or does not lie, on a spectrum. Early identification is a noble aim but moves us into uncharted waters. Until it can be shown that doing so carries a real value and/or that biological markers can offer firmer validation, expanding the range of this diagnosis has more risks than benefits.

Chapter 8

Bipolar and Related Disorders

BIPOLAR DISORDERS IN DSM-5

Kraepelin was the first psychiatrist to systematically describe manic-depressive illness. Later another German expert, Karl Leonhard (1979), suggested a name change to *bipolar disorder*, distinguishing between cases of mood disorder presenting with depressive episodes (unipolar) and those that swing from depression to mania (bipolar). Eventually, bipolar disorder itself was divided into two types, one with full mania (bipolar-I) and the other with hypomania (bipolar-II; Parker, 2012).

The criteria for bipolar-I disorder have not been changed in the new manual. The patient must meet criteria for a manic episode, and the clinician must specify whether there are psychotic features, mixed features, catatonic features, rapid cycling, anxiety, suicide risk, a seasonal pattern, or a post partum onset. For bipolar-II disorder, there must have been a hypomanic episode, as well as a history of major depressive episodes, and symptoms must be clinically significant.

Bipolar-I disorder with classical manic episodes is one of the best-defined illnesses in the DSM manual. Even so, there are problems with its boundaries. The category of schizo-affective disorder allows clinicians to fudge the question as to whether a patient has schizophrenia or a mood disorder. Years ago, Pope and Lipinski (1978) showed that most of these cases can be placed in bipolar disorder or schizophrenia by taking a careful family history and examining treatment response. Later, Lake and Hurwitz (2006) concluded that most schizo-affective patients have a mood disorder and are simply showing more severe psychotic features than clinicians expect. But this diagnosis is sometimes used to describe schizophrenic patients who are depressed. Contrary to clinical lore, schizophrenia is not necessarily associated with flattened affect; many patients are understandably depressed about living with a disabling mental disorder (Andreasen, 1979). DSM-5 might have removed the schizo-affective category entirely but chose not to do so.

The other disorders described in this chapter of DSM-5 are rare. Cyclothymic disorder describes subthreshold hypomanic and depressive symptoms over a 2-year course. Unspecified bipolar disorder (previously bipolar NOS) is rarely used but could become common, as it allows clinicians to diagnose the disorder even when symptoms do not meet the threshold for either bipolar-I or bipolar-II. As we will see, the research literature is replete with studies that call such cases "bipolar-II" (despite the absence of hypomania), consistent with the concept of a bipolar spectrum.

THE OVERDIAGNOSIS OF BIPOLAR DISORDER

In the past, bipolar disorder was underdiagnosed and was often confused with schizophrenia. Forty years ago, the use of lithium for the acute treatment of mania, and for the prevention of relapse, changed everything. These results led psychiatrists to wonder if they might get the same results in other patients by reconsidering whether patients in other categories actually suffer from a form of bipolar disorder. Schizophrenia was the first target for rediagnosis. For example, abnormal states of excitement previously categorized as catatonic schizophrenia could be redefined as forms of mania. "First-rank" symptoms of schizophrenia (such as thought broadcasting and thought insertion, long thought to be pathognomonic of schizophrenia) turned out to be common in manic patients (Abrams & Taylor, 1981). The most convincing evidence for changes in diagnosis was the observation that some patients previously diagnosed with schizophrenia could be treated successfully with lithium.

Because lithium, unlike antipsychotics, also did a good job of preventing relapses of mania, psychiatrists were keen to use it, and many more psychotic patients began to be diagnosed with bipolar disorder (Paris, 2009). But this change in practice had shallow roots. Rediagnosis could be right or wrong, but there was no way of telling. Most clinicians looked to see whether patients got better on lithium. But it is often hard to determine whether a patient has responded to this drug, given that bipolar disorder is episodic and that lithium is often prescribed during a hospital admission—at the same time as numerous other interventions. The diagnosis usually becomes clearer when patients are followed over time.

There has been much controversy about the boundaries of bipolar-II (Parker, 2012). The introduction of this category in DSM-IV, with mood swinging from depression to hypomania, was a good decision, since typical cases are often seen, but bipolar-II has become too popular for its own good. We have seen a diagnostic epidemic, largely because of a preference for identifying conditions that can be managed with drugs. It has also opened the door to a major expansion of the bipolar diagnosis, so that all phenomena marked by mood instability can be seen as reflecting milder forms of bipolarity on a spectrum. Bipolarity came to be defined in ways that expand into the boundaries of other mental disorders, and some have claimed it is present in a large percentage of the patients who see psychiatrists (Akiskal et al., 2006). Strict observance of criteria would lead these cases to be diagnosed as bipolar-NOS, or as other mental disorders.

Kraepelin (1921) suggested that milder forms of mania can develop in the absence of classical symptoms. But he probably would have been surprised to see physicians diagnosing bipolar disorder in 5% to 10% of the general population. In recent years, any and all forms of mood swings or unstable moods have been proposed to lie on a spectrum (Akiskal, 2002; Angst & Gamma, 2002). This tendency to see mood disorders, personality disorders, and impulsive disorders as "bipolar" has spread rapidly. It has even entered common parlance. And the concept has been expanded to include an even broader group of clinical problems.

The leaders of the bipolar spectrum movement have been an American psychiatrist, Hagop Akiskal (2002), and a Swiss psychiatrist, Jules Angst (1998), supported by other prominent researchers (Goodwin & Jamison, 2008; Ghaemi et al., 2002). All claim that bipolarity is much more prevalent than previously believed. In light of their suggestion that up to 40% of all psychiatric patients suffer from the condition, I have described them as "bipolar imperialists" (Paris, 2009).

To explain my critique, let us return to the traditional definition of mania based on a "triad" of signs and symptoms: elevated affect, psychomotor excitement, and racing thoughts. Classically, psychiatrists did not diagnose mania in the absence of euphoria. However, soon after the introduction of lithium, it was observed that bipolar-I patients can show irritability rather than elevated mood and that this symptom can also respond to mood stabilizers (Winokur & Tsuang, 1975). That observation led some to question whether states of excitement, irritability, and aggression seen in other categories of mental disorder could be symptoms of mania and whether the classical triad is a necessary condition for bipolarity. The clinical situation was further modified by the concept of a "mixed episode," a poorly researched category in which patients seem both depressed and irritable. (This clinical picture corresponds to what used to be called "agitated depression.") In DSM-5, such episodes will be a specifier rather than a separate diagnosis.

The key issue in making a bipolar-II diagnosis is to ensure that patients meet criteria for hypomania. These episodes have quite specific requirements related to time scale and persistence. A hypomanic episode, as defined in DSM-IV-TR, consisted of "persistently elevated, expansive, or irritable mood, lasting throughout at least 4 days." If not directly observed, the assessment of hypomania by retrospective patient report is difficult, as one cannot readily determine whether mood elevation was persistent or how long it lasted (Dunner & Tay, 1993). Brief periods of elevated mood that do not persist describe mood instability but do not meet formal criteria for hypomania. They can also be mimicked by substance use, most particularly stimulants.

Enthusiasts of the bipolar spectrum object to the 4-day rule, which is why they so often conflate bipolar-NOS with bipolar-II. One could dimensionalize hypomania so that symptoms for the full 4 days would not be required. But scale and timing are often used in medicine to establish boundaries between pathology and normality. Before introducing a spectrum concept that would lead to major changes in psychiatric diagnosis, we should know whether mood swings share a common psychopathological mechanism.

The definition of hypomania is crucial. Admittedly, the DSM-IV requirement that elated or irritable mood be present continuously for at least 4 days is arbitrary. The problem is that a shorter period would be equally arbitrary. Some patients with personality disorders can have mood swings lasting only an hour or so. Clinical assessment also has to be done carefully to determine that hypomania has been continuous for 4 days. Even more important, mood swings that are primarily subjective and do not lead to changes in behavior that other people are almost sure to notice (rapid speech, little need for sleep, overspending) are not diagnostic of hypomania. Removing this requirement would have vast implications for diagnosis and treatment.

Benazzi (2004) recommended that a day or two of continuously feeling "high" be sufficient to identify hypomania. Angst (1998) argued that patients with 2-day "hypomania" should be considered to be bipolar, particularly if confirmed by family history and/or long-term outcome. I do not disagree that such cases exist or that bipolar disorder can begin with subclinical symptoms. But it does not follow that *all* patients with these features fall within the bipolar spectrum. This is the same problem we saw with attenuated psychosis syndrome—it produces too many false–positives.

Moreover, because most information about hypomania is collected retrospectively, it is difficult to be sure that abnormal mood has persisted without respite for the entire period. Lowering the bar would inevitably lead to a huge increase in diagnosis of bipolar disorder. Actually, this has already happened. Few clinicians observe the 4-day rule but respond with a "bipolar" knee-jerk to mood swings of any kind. The result is the prescription of mood stabilizers and antipsychotics to patients who may or may not need them.

In the end, DSM-5 did not modify the 4-day rule for hypomania. Most senior people in the field concluded that the evidence was not strong enough to do so, and the consequences would be unpredictable. This was a reassuringly sensible decision.

Ghaemi et al. (2002) proposed a category of bipolar-III to describe hypomania brought on by antidepressants. DSM-IV did not consider this a separate syndrome but an effect of a drug. In DSM-5, episodes of mania or hypomania that follow treatment with antidepressants are classified in the same way as other cases—assuming they continue well beyond the original pharmacological intervention.

Actually the scenario of a shift to hypomania after antidepressant therapy is rare. Confusion arises because bipolar disorder often emerges from an initial depression, and a switch can be independent of drug treatment (Parker & Parker, 2003). Interpreting the emergence of mania as *caused* by an antidepressant, rather than as an evolution of a disease process, may be illusory. This makes it doubtful whether we need a diagnosis of bipolar-III.

Ghaemi et al. (2002) also proposed adding a category of bipolar-IV that would describe ultra-rapid mood swings, even those that only last for a few hours. These clinical phenomena are better described as affective instability and may not be a form of bipolarity at all, as they are frequent in patients with personality disorders (Koenigsberg, 2010). The very use of the term "ultra-rapid" conflates rapid-cycling bipolar illness, defined by frequently recurring episodes of mania or hypomania, with mood that changes from day to day or from hour to hour. Thus affective instability, brief mood changes characterized by temporal instability, high intensity, and delayed recovery from dysphoric states could be an entirely different psychopathological phenomenon. Without biological markers, how can we know?

Once ultra-rapid mood swings are admitted as diagnostic criteria, many other mental disorders would fall within the bipolar spectrum. Again, these concepts depend entirely on phenomenological resemblances that are observable but ultimately superficial. We should not assume that common symptoms reflect similar underlying disease processes. Mood instability is a common symptom that can be seen in many conditions, including personality disorders (where it is a primary feature), substance abuse disorders, and eating disorders. Akiskal (2002) takes this as evidence that *all* of these patients are "really" bipolar. Making affective instability equivalent to bipolarity has also led some child psychiatrists (e.g., Chang, 2007) to redefine many of the common behavior disorders of childhood as "pediatric bipolar disorder."

Definitional problems have also affected estimates of how common bipolar disorder is in the community. In the Epidemiological Catchment Area study (Robins & Regier, 1991), the lifetime prevalence of bipolar-I was 0.8%, and bipolar-II was 0.5%. These were conservative and believable numbers. But in the National Comorbidity Study (Kessler et al., 1995), the lifetime prevalence of bipolar-I went up to 1.6%. Then, the National Comorbidity Study Replication reported the combined prevalence for bipolar-I and bipolar-II to be 3.9% (Kessler et al., 2005), an increase that followed from a looser definition of hypomania. All these numbers were based on DSM-IV criteria. When "subclinical" symptoms such as mood instability and irritability are assessed with a new instrument to determine the frequency of bipolar spectrum disorders (Merikangas et al., 2007), bipolar-I was estimated to have a prevalence of 1%, bipolar II went up to 1.1% (already a notable increase), and subthreshold cases added an additional 2.4%, for a total of 4.5%.

Depending on how much you broaden the spectrum, community prevalence could be even higher: Angst (1998) published an estimate of 8%, twice as high as even the most elevated numbers. In clinical samples, where protocols can be designed to identify spectrum symptoms using dimensional "indexes" of bipolarity, prevalence can be even more dramatically elevated. For example, 39% of *all* patients in a large study of patients at multiple sites in France were reported to have experienced episodes of broadly defined hypomania (Akiskal et al., 2006).

The problem is the absence of a gold standard. The psychiatrists who want to expand DSM criteria conduct research using scales designed to measure what they call "soft bipolarity"—that is, spectrum cases defined by putative subthreshold symptoms. But how do we know that these subthreshold symptoms are true indicators of bipolarity? Phenomenological resemblances are not sufficient. It is possible that subclinical symptoms of moodiness reflect a different type of psychopathology—or normal variations not necessarily related to mood disorders.

The concept of a bipolar spectrum stands on firmer ground when applied to recurrent unipolar depression. Here we have a problem with *underdiagnosis* of bipolarity. Kraepelin (1921) was the first to observe that severe depression can develop over time into bipolar disorder. This outcome is more likely to occur in the presence of an early onset, a recurrent course, atypical symptomatology, and a family history of bipolarity (Benazzi, 2002).

Every practitioner will have seen such cases. But the frequency of this outcome in outpatient practice or primary care has been exaggerated. As the concept became popularized, I received many consultations from family doctors asking whether patients with *mild to moderate* depression, who have not responded to drug therapy, were "really bipolar." Patients, who can be attracted to faddish diagnoses, may also adopt this point of view, breezily stating that they (or their relatives and friends) have a bipolar illness. Expanding the bipolar spectrum has also been supported by the media (who like a simple story) and by the pharmaceutical industry (which is looking for a larger market).

The promoters of the bipolar spectrum are sincere but misguided. They are promoting models that lead to a large number of false–positive diagnoses. They want to rediagnose a very large number of patients in psychiatry and put them on mood stabilizers and/or antipsychotics. A broad bipolar spectrum would take up a very large chunk of psychiatry, but the fad is based on enthusiasm rather than on evidence.

One way to validate diagnoses is by identifying a characteristic treatment response. The concept of "pharmacological dissection" is based on evidence that the same agent can produce the same effect in patients fall in different categories (Klein, 1987). Although classical bipolar disorder usually responds to mood stabilizers, we lack randomized clinical trials to show whether these drugs work in the same way in spectrum disorders and the evidence suggests they don't (Paris, 2012). Patients with putative bipolarity do not consistently respond to the pharmacotherapy that works in classical cases (Patten & Paris, 2008).

For example, in patients with personality disorders associated with affective instability, the evidence for using *any* drug for these clinical populations is quite weak (Paris, 2008c; Kendall et al., 2009), and mood stabilizers cannot be considered to be standard treatment. Confusion arises because psychiatric drugs can have broad sedative effects that reduce the frequency of all kinds of problematic symptoms and behaviors. No one would claim that relief from pain obtained by prescribing analgesics proves that all patients who respond to them have the same illness.

PEDIATRIC BIPOLAR DISORDER

In recent years, controversy has arisen as to whether bipolarity can be diagnosed in pre-pubertal children. Since the time of Kraepelin (1921), it had been generally accepted that bipolar disorder rarely begins before adolescence. And although no one disagrees that classical bipolarity can be seen shortly after puberty, the concept of a bipolar spectrum has led clinicians to diagnose it in adolescents who would be better described as having a personality disorder (Chanen et al., 2008). There has also been confusion about concepts, because for some "childhood" means before age 18 years, whereas for others it means before adolescence.

The concept that mania can begin in childhood and is actually common before puberty, has become influential but controversial (Wozniak, 2005; Faedda et al., 2004). Frances (2010f), who views pediatric bipolar disorder as an example of a diagnostic fad, commented:

"To become a fad, a psychiatric diagnosis requires 3 preconditions: a pressing need, an engaging story, and influential prophets. The pressing need arises from the fact that disturbed and disturbing kids are very often encountered in clinical, school, and correctional settings. They suffer and cause suffering to those around them—making themselves noticeable to families, doctors, and teachers. Everyone feels enormous pressure to do something. Previous diagnoses (especially conduct or oppositional disorder) provided little hope and no call to action. In contrast, a diagnosis of childhood Bipolar Disorder creates a justification for medication and for expanded school services. The medications have broad and nonspecific effects that are often helpful in reducing anger, even if the diagnosis is inaccurate."

What is actually observed in so-called "bipolar children"? If you read the research reports carefully, they describe broad and persistent emotional dysregulation (Geller et al., 2008; Birmaher et al., 2009). Although these children have mood swings, they do not develop manic or hypomanic episodes. They are moody, irritable, oppositional, and likely to misbehave—like all children with disruptive behavior disorders. Their grandiose thinking usually consists of little beyond boastfulness.

No evidence from genetics, neurobiology, follow-up studies or treatment response shows that this syndrome has anything in common with classical bipolarity. In a recent prospective study of the children of bipolar parents (Duffy et al., 2009), mood disorder episodes (mostly depression) started only after puberty, and no features of bipolarity were observed in the cohort prior to that. Another prospective study found that children of bipolar parents are at risk for ADHD rather than bipolarity (Birmaher et al., 2010).

Some of the evidence for this theory has been based on follow-up studies of a group of children in St. Louis (Geller et al., 2008). Yet this research group did *not* find that the syndrome evolves into bipolar disorder in adolescence, and others have also failed to find such a relationship (Birmaher & Axelson, 2006). Although the clinical picture can persist over many years (Geller et al., 2002), it remains at the level of "soft bipolarity." Although these children show moodiness and irritability, they do not have hypomanic episodes. In the end, symptoms considered to be "bipolar" in adults need not have the same meaning in children. Moodiness and disruptive behavior are very common among children studied in community surveys (Duffy, 2007). They are also among the most frequent symptoms in children referred to psychiatrists.

Brotman et al. (2006) introduced a different term to describe these cases: *severe mood dysregulation* (SMD). They also found that children with this picture go on to develop depression—*not* mania—later in life. Similar ideas have been proposed by others (Carlson et al., 2010; Leibenluft, 2011). DSM-5 at one point suggested using the term "temper dysregulation disorder," but because that diagnosis could be confused with temper tantrums, it was replaced by *disruptive mood dysregulation disorder* (DMDD). This terminology views the syndrome as a variant of a mood disorder, not as a classical behavior disorder such as conduct disorder or oppositional defiant disorder. One purpose of this new terminology could be to discourage an automatic prescription of mood stabilizers and antipsychotics. However, the wish to prescribe drugs to seriously disturbed children does not only depend on diagnosis. No one would be surprised if children with DMDD routinely receive antipsychotics.

Finally, "pediatric bipolar disorder" has a large overlap with other diagnoses. Geller et al. (2008) observed particularly strong comorbidity with disruptive behavioral disorders (conduct disorder, oppositional defiant disorder, and attention-deficit hyperactivity disorder [ADHD]). None of those conditions are precursors of adult bipolarity. Long-term studies following children with ADHD into adulthood (Weiss & Hechtman, 1993; Manuzza & Klein, 2000), as well as of children with conduct disorder (Zoccolillo et al., 1992), have shown an increased risk for developing antisocial personality disorder and substance use, *not* for bipolar disorder.

This problem of whether to extend the bipolar spectrum to children is not just theoretical. There are important clinical consequences, as shown by the dramatic increase in the prescription of antipsychotic drugs to children—including preschool children (Olfson et al., 2010). That trend has been most striking in the United States but has also spread to Great Britain (Rani et al., 2008).

Psychiatry has received criticism, both fair and unfair, for its use of drugs. But when we give neuroleptics to patients with schizophrenia or mood stabilizers to patients with adult bipolar disorder, we know that the consequences of leaving the illness untreated are more severe than any side effects these agents may produce. In contrast, when we give drugs to young children seen as bipolar, we do not have the same evidence base and do not know the long-term consequences.

Thus the diagnosis of bipolar disorder in children has the potential to do harm, by encouraging overly aggressive pharmacological treatment. DSM-5, to its credit, is trying to recognize the problem by not calling these cases "bipolar." Even so, the diagnosis of DMDD will probably run into the same difficulties. Child psychiatry, once noted for its interest in family life and social issues, has become focused on biological mechanisms and pharmacological solutions. These problems are made worse by seeing almost every symptom as a reflection of abnormal mood.

In summary, DSM-5, faced with demands for expanding the bipolar spectrum, has acceded in some areas but held firm in others. Even so, the increase in bipolar diagnosis has already had a profound effect on practice (Yutzy et al., 2012). Only time will tell how future generations will look back on the current practice of prescribing mood stabilizers and antipsychotics to so many patients. In 50 years, it might not be seen as a breakthrough but as a harmful fad.

Chapter 9

Depressive Disorders

Almost everyone recognizes the experience of feeling depressed, and moodiness is almost universal. Because these experiences are so common, we need to critically examine the boundaries of mood disorders. How does depression differ from sadness? How does bipolar disorder differ from common moodiness? Is depression always a disorder in its own right, or can it be a symptom of another condition? The problem for DSM-5 was whether to be restrictive or expansive in defining what constitutes a disorder.

WHAT IS DEPRESSION?

Since the time of Hippocrates, *melancholia* has been recognized as a medical illness. In the past, psychiatrists saw this clinical picture as qualitatively different from milder forms of depression (Parker, 2011). Melancholia lasts weeks to months, during which patients suffer from despondency, irritability, and restlessness, with a slowing down of mental processes and movement, diminished appetite, sleeplessness, and powerful suicidal urges. Mood is clearly disproportionate to external stressors and associated with psychomotor retardation or agitation, severe cognitive impairment, prominent vegetative symptoms, and/or psychosis (Parker, 2011).

This is a different picture from "garden-variety" depression. As psychiatrists have long been taught, depression can be a symptom, a syndrome, or a disorder. The concept that depression is one condition, varying only in severity, has obscured these important distinctions, Prospective studies find that up to half of the population, and possibly more, will experience changes in mood that meet DSM-IV criteria for a major depressive episode at some time during their lives (Moffitt et al., 2010). And those data come from a study that has followed people only in their 30s. Parker (2005) noted that other prospective data have suggested that almost 80% of the population experiences a major depression during their lifetime. The numbers could easily go up to 100% with the diluting of exclusions for normal reactions such as grief (Wakefield et al., 2007). Obviously, the problem is diagnostic inflation resulting from loose definitions.

Some view these findings as confirming that depression is the "common cold of psychiatry." Alternatively, the current definition of major depression may be seriously over-inclusive, in that it fails to distinguish between problems of living and mental disorder. This conclusion is supported by research in the community showing that bereavement, whether simple or complicated, is not associated with the wide range of symptoms that characterize classical major depression (Gilman et al., 2012).

The separation of psychotic and neurotic depression in DSM-I and DSM-II was an attempt, however misguided, to address these distinctions. It considered a psychotic (and/or melancholic) picture to be "endogenous," whereas a neurotic depression was seen as primarily environmental in origin. But that separation was invalid. People with psychotic depression can fall ill after being exposed to stressors, and people with milder forms of depression may also be biologically prone to mood disorders. Thus depression cannot be subclassified on the basis of etiological factors that are highly complex and interactive. But we are still left with the question—is depression one disorder or many?

THE UNITARY THEORY OF DEPRESSION

Forty years ago, in an influential review paper, Akiskal and McKinney (1973) proposed that all depressions lie on a continuum, differing only in severity. They noted that distinctions cannot be made on the basis of unproven etiological theories and that symptoms, family history, outcome, and treatment response tend to cut across all forms of depression.

The unitary theory was adopted in DSM-III and has held sway since. A "major depressive episode" is diagnosed if patients meet five of nine listed criteria for a minimum of 2 weeks. Severe cases can then be sub-typed as psychotic or melancholic. Although the unitary theory became a conventional wisdom, it continues to be challenged on the grounds that melancholia is different from garden-variety depression (Parker, 2005). The assumption that these are degrees of the same illness remains questionable.

A second, and more serious problem with the unitary theory is that it does not separate psychopathology from normal unhappiness (Horwitz & Wakefield, 2007). The DSM definition is so broad that it is hard to imagine anyone who has not met criteria at some point of their life.

An overly short time scale is the most important source of over-diagnosis. How easy is it, after a loss or serious setback in life, to be depressed for 2 weeks at a time? Given the evidence that most cases of mild depression remit rapidly (Patten, 2008), 4 weeks to 6 weeks would have provided a more valid cut-off, as would recurrence and chronicity.

A third issue is just how "major" is major depression. DSM requires patients to meet five criteria. But nobody knows where the number five came from, except that it is more than half of nine. Moreover, a diag-nosis can be made on the basis of milder symptoms alone: a low mood plus loss of interest or pleasure, loss of energy, reduced concentration, and insomnia. All these features occur in transitory mood states related to environmental stressors (Horwitz & Wakefield, 2007; Patten, 2008). Although research on the DSM-IV criteria in community populations does not find a clear cut-off from normality (Kendler & Gardner, 1998), the criteria for major depression are quite heterogeneous, with some recent studies (Lux & Kendler, 2010; Lux et al., 2010) showing that a mixture of cognitive and neurovegetative criteria does not provide a valid basis for rating severity.

If previous editions of DSM had required more than five criteria, that would also have helped to define depression in a valid way. It would also have been useful to have criteria that *must* be present, rather than mixing and matching like a menu at a Chinese restaurant. As it stands, the only required feature among the nine is low mood itself (or a loss of interest and pleasure). The bar is set too low, and scoring severity does not really address the problem. For example, subclinical cases with four or even fewer symptoms are also distressed. Yet one could say much the same about three, two, or even one symptom.

Finally, because even a seven-digit phone number is too long to be remembered by most people unless written down, clinicians do not actually remember nine criteria in making a diagnosis. Zimmerman et al. (2011) found that simplifying the criteria list to five criteria rather than nine: low mood, loss of interest, guilt or worthlessness, impaired concentration or indecisiveness, and death wishes or suicidal thoughts, of which three would be required to make the diagnosis, gives the much the same result as DSM-IV. Even so, simplifying an algorithim does not address the question as to whether depression is too broadly defined. Parker et al. (2010) proposed an alternative procedure, in which psychotic, melancholic, and non-melancholic types are immediately identified, rather than being after-thoughts to an overall diagnosis of major depression. This was designed to encourage clinicians to recognize psychotic and melancholic depressions, which require different methods of treatment and respond differently to therapy as unique.

In summary, 40 years after Akiskal and McKinney, we still cannot conclude that severe, moderate, and mild depression are points on a single spectrum, or separate syndromes. As we will see, major depression is a heterogeneous diagnosis that can mislead clinicians about treatment of patients. There is no real clinical value in overidentifying depression.

EXCLUSIONS FOR DIAGNOSIS

Should depression be diagnosed if a stressor is present that would make almost anyone unhappy? DSM-IV allowed for the exclusion of extended periods of symptomatic distress following bereavement but did not apply the same rule to other losses. Life events such as divorce or job loss can also produce symptoms that resemble grief. Depressive symptoms, whether caused by bereavement or by other life stressors, are similar, and excluding grief helps to distinguish the normal from the pathological (Wakefield & First, 2012). Why not extend the exclusions to recognize that when people suffer losses, they can be expected to have transient depressive symptoms?

DSM-5 has moved in the opposite direction. Initially it wanted to remove the grief exclusion entirely—once again expanding the range of diagnosis. This is another example of inflating mental disorder so that it enters the realm of normality. It also shows a failure to account for the social context in which symptoms develop. Grief produces symptoms that are similar to depression, but that does not prove they are one and the same. Moreover separating grief from depression allows clinicians to describe patients with different outcomes and different treatment needs (Parker et al., 2011). Kleinman (2012), an expert in psychiatric anthropology, expressed his disagreement by describing in print how his grief for the recent death of his wife could be diagnosed as a major depression.

Wakefield and First (2012) have proposed a solution that would involve raising the bar for severity and determining the extent to which symptoms are contextual. The fact that some patients remain depressed several months after bereavement could be taken into account by rewriting the criteria. Thus those who have 2 weeks of depressive symptoms after a loss would be diagnosed as having a normal reaction, whereas those who suffer for extended periods could still be diagnosed with a major depression. This is close to the solution eventually adopted by DSM-5 in May 2012, in which clinicians are warned not to diagnose major depression if grief, even if prolonged, best accounts for symptoms. It also provides a category, for now relegated to the Appendix, called "persistent complex bereavement disorder."

The removal of the bereavement exclusion would have meant that many more patients would be diagnosed with, and treated for, depression. Perhaps this has already happened—many people take antidepressants without any diagnosis (Mojtabai & Olfson, 2011). Wakefield (2010b) has suggested that diagnostic expansiveness reflects the nature of today's outpatient practice, and psychiatrists do not want to be limited to severe disorders but want diagnoses to justify treating whatever problems they see. Perhaps doing so would make little difference if treatment mainly consisted of counseling or psychotherapy. But the diagnosis of major depression leads physicians to prescribe drugs—despite the evidence that less severe cases do not consistently respond at more than a placebo level (Kirsch et al., 2008). And once patients are put on antidepressants, clinicians are afraid to stop them, for fear of a relapse.

Fortunately, most antidepressants are not very toxic, even when taken on a long-term basis. But the diagnostic system should not encourage physicians to prescribe drugs that may or may not work and that patients go on taking for years. Recent data have shown that *11%* of all Americans over age 12 years are taking an antidepressant (Pratt et al., 2011). Psychiatry and primary care have come to see unhappiness as a mental disorder.

Epidemiological research, if based on DSM criteria, tends to support the idea that depression is ubiquitous. In the National Comorbidity Survey, a large-scale epidemiological study, lifetime prevalence was 16.6% (Kessler et al., 2005). Even these numbers could be an underestimate. Forgetting about a depressive episode once it resolves is generally adaptive. Thus researchers using prospective rather than retrospective data (Moffitt et al., 2009) have found when one accounts for the episodes that have been forgotten, up to half of all individuals in the general population meet criteria at some point in their life up to age 32 years.

But community studies of depression include many mild cases that do not require medical treatment (Patten, 2008). Thus, there is little point in screening to move people into the mental health system (Patten, 2008). The problem of false–positives casts a shadow on all epidemiological studies of mood disorders. Enthusiasm for antidepressant treatment has led to the idea, supported by mental health associations, of screening the general population to diagnose all forms of depression including subthreshold cases. This would have the unfortunate effect of shifting the focus of psychiatry from severely ill patients, who we are already hard pressed to treat properly, to normal people who have transient episodes of depression from which they will recover. Even if depression is the common cold of psychiatry, a cold should not be confused with pneumonia.

The unitary theory, incorporated into the DSM system, arose from a specific *theory* about mood disorders, consistent with the tendency of DSM to see all mental illness as biological and on a continuum with normality. Yet none of the current categories of depression reflect unique pathological processes or endophenotypes. Even in melancholia, which can sometimes be associated with endocrinological changes (Parker et al., 2010), biological markers are not consistent enough to be used to validate diagnosis. And in mild to moderate depression, we have no markers at all.

Current mood disorder categories fail to help clinicians select specific treatment methods, which in any case requires more than a simple diagnosis. The unitary concept of major depression is a poor guide to therapy, because patients are heterogeneous, and drug responses are unpredictable in non-melancholic depression. Healy (2009) has even spoken of the *creation* of major depression, given that the category is not well validated and not always all that "major."

DSM-III addressed variations in clinical presentation by allowing additional codes for severity within the broader diagnosis of major depression. But it is one thing to include these options in the manual and another to get clinicians to use them. What seems to have happened is that treatments designed for melancholic depression are being applied to depression of any kind (Paris, 2010).

The editors of DSM-III had, at one point, considered introducing a category of "minor depression" to describe less severe symptoms. In the end, that category fell into a larger wastebasket—mood disorder, not otherwise specified. Patients with transient symptoms who do not meet five criteria for major depression for 2 weeks can also be diagnosed with an "adjustment disorder with depressed mood," but that diagnosis is not widely utilized. Finally, patients with chronic but subclinical symptoms can be diagnosed with "dysthymia," if they meet only two criteria (present most of the time over a 2-year period). Although clinicians often see patients with dysthymia, it is a poorly researched category, which could include milder mood disorders and/or depressed feelings associated with many other diagnoses, most particularly personality disorders, and these cases do not respond consistently to antidepressants (Klein and Santiago, 2003).

CHANGES IN DSM-5

In light of all these unresolved problems, it is reassuring to see a relatively light level of revision in DSM-5. As in previous editions of the manual, a major depressive episode still requires the presence of five of nine criteria (low mood, loss of interest, weight loss or gain, insomnia or hypersomnia, psychomotor agitation or retardation, worthlessness, reduced concentration, and thoughts of death), accompanied by clinically significant distress. Then a major depressive disorder (single episode or recurrent) can be diagnosed. Dysthymia has been renamed "chronic depressive disorder," which combines cases in which patients retain subthreshold symptoms over a 2-year period.

It has long been known that anxiety and depression cannot readily be separated and often, if not usually, found in the same patients (Goldberg & Goodyer, 2005). One proposed change in DSM-5 was for a comorbid anxiety dimension, plus the addition of a new disorder, called mixed anxiety-depression (three symptoms of major depression plus two of anxiety). Wakefield (2012) expressed concern about the low bar set for this diagnosis. The proposal was dropped in 2012, when it did not prove reliable in clinical trials.

A second change concerns the definition of mixed episodes (in which depression and mania can be found in the same patient at the same time). The manual offers a "mixed features" specifier applicable to manic, hypomanic, and major depressive episodes. This change allows clinicians to score subthreshold symptoms, making it more likely that mixed episodes will be identified. That may or may not be a useful idea.

A third change is the option of scoring severity dimensions for major depressive episodes. This procedure depends on an unweighted symptom count—based on instruments using self-report like the Patient Health Questionnaire-9 (PHQ-9; Kroenke et al., 2001) or clinical ratings, like the Clinical Global Impression (CGI; Guy, 1976). Scoring symptoms formally could have advantages over clinical impressions of severity but is not really that objective, because clinical judgments still have to be made.

The fourth change is that DSM-5 has moved the category of pre-menstrual dysphoric disorder from the appendix of DSM-IV into the mood disorders section of the manual. Premenstrual dysphoric disorder had been moved from the appendix to the main manual and lists 11 possible symptoms, of which 5 have to be present (associated with clinically significant distress). The list describes mood swings and irritability that occur during most cycles and that remit when menstruation occurs. This disorder had been considered for inclusion in DSM-IV but was eventually relegated to an appendix. The concern was that common symptoms that many women experience could be medicalized. The rationale behind the change is that, as has been known for some time, this syndrome can be treated effectively with antidepressants (Steiner et al., 1995). However, two concerns remain. One is the potential stigmatization of women. The other is that the diagnostic criteria are too easily met, leading to unnecessary pharmacological treatment in patients whose symptoms are mild. This is another example of a problem that afflicts DSM-5 as a whole.

Finally, disruptive mood dysregulation disorder, a category that applies to children ages 6 years to 18 years, has been added. Because this condition has a number of features in common with disruptive behavior disorders, it will be discussed in Chapter 13.

First (2011) reviewed the changes in DSM-5 in the light of a cost–benefit analysis. He expressed concern about false–positives (i.e., diagnosing patients who are unhappy with depression) and about clinical utility and problematic implementation, given that busy clinicians are unlikely to carry out complex scoring that might best be reserved for researchers. As with so many other revisions in the manual, the changes in mood disorders have not been subjected to the kind of detailed testing needed to determine what effect they will have on practice.

IMPLICATIONS OF DIAGNOSIS FOR TREATMENT

In contemporary medicine, clinicians often assume that *any* patient meeting DSM criteria for major depression has to be put on antidepressants. Some physicians are afraid of lawsuits if they don't order these agents. The fact that the diagnosis exists and that the drugs have a name suggesting they counter-depression is sufficient for a knee-jerk prescription. Few follow the British guidelines published by the National Institute of Clinical Excellence (NICE, 2007), which sensibly recommended that physicians watch and wait for a few weeks before putting patients with mild to moderate depression on any drugs.

The adoption of a single category of major depression is an important support for the idea that all cases require similar treatment. Yet when compared to placebo, severe depression responds much more consistently to antidepressants than mild to moderate symptoms (Kirsch et al., 2008; Shelton & Fawcett, 2010). Although other meta-analyses (e.g., Gibbon et al., 2012) have supported a wider response, we should be humbled by these research findings. They show that antidepressants, however useful, are not consistently superior to placebo in producing remissions in patients with less severe symptoms. (This is a general principle in medicine: treatment response is easier to measure in the presence of severity.) Placebo effects are low in severe depression, but strong enough in milder depressions to closely match the efficacy of drugs. These differences in response based on initial severity have long been observed (Elkin et al., 1989). Although drugs are almost always necessary in severe depression, psychotherapy is just as effective in milder cases. These differential treatment effects tend to support the conclusion that "major depression" is a heterogeneous condition and not one diagnosis with varying levels of severity (Parker, 2005).

The unitary theory of major depression also underlies the concept of "treatment-resistant depression" (i.e., the scenario in which depressive symptoms do not respond well to drug treatment). This concept, based on the idea that depression *should* respond, has led to a wide use of augmentation and switching strategies. Some of these procedures can be useful, but much recent research, particularly the STAR-D effectiveness study (Valenstein, 2006; Rush et al., 2006) has suggested antidepressants are useful but greatly overrated. About two-thirds of patients eventually recover from depression with treatment, but many will recover with time alone.

In summary, a diagnosis of major depression is, by itself, a poor guide to practice. Inconsistent efficacy of treatment occurs because drugs are being prescribed to a heterogeneous group, some of whom have a true mental disorder, and some of whom are just unhappy.

In the history of medicine, physicians have expressly aimed to treat disease on the basis of a detailed understanding of the mechanisms behind pathology. But just as often, physicians develop cures and only then go in search of diseases. We should be cautious about rushing to offer panacea-like treatments and to justify this practice by creating overly broad diagnostic categories. Depression remains a central focus of clinical practice but is classified in a broad and misleading way that fails to distinguish between cases that require pharmacotherapy and those that may not. The result is overdiagnosis and overtreatment.

Chapter 10

Anxiety Disorders, Trauma, and the Obsessive-Compulsive Spectrum

Anxiety is as universal as sadness. There are many things to fear in life, and *not* worrying about them would be a mistake. So at what point can one say that anxiety is pathological? Although the usual guideline is that emotions are excessive if they cause dysfunction, the boundary between normal and pathological anxiety can be arbitrary (Horwitz & Wakefield, 2012).

Anxiety is a psychological experience, separated from syndromes with prominent physical symptoms. Yet it has long been known that internalizing disorders often present with unexplained physical distress, particularly in specific cultures and social settings (Gone & Kirmayer, 2010). This may account for the overlap between anxiety and physical symptoms (Simms et al., 2012). Also, in clinical settings, anxiety and depression often co-exist. One of the most common presentations of psychological distress in primary care is a mixture of both types of symptoms (Goldberg & Goodyer, 2005). It is not known which is primary, which is secondary, or whether both are manifestations of a common process.

Although there is symptomatic overlap among anxiety disorders, post-traumatic stress disorder (PTSD), and obsessive-compulsive disorder (OCD), these conditions have a different clinical presentation and are now separate chapters in the DSM manual. (This chapter will discuss all three.) Even so, separation into categories on the basis of overt symptoms may not be fully valid, given that family members of a patient with one anxiety disorder can have another (Bienvenu et al., 2011). Research on community populations shows a strong overlap between *all* syndromes related to anxiety and internalization (Tambs et al., 2009).

PANIC DISORDER AND GENERALIZED ANXIETY DISORDER

DSM-IV described five forms of anxiety disorder (panic, generalized anxiety disorder [GAD], OCD, phobia, and PTSD), two of which have now been moved into other groupings. It may be worth looking back in history to see how all these distinctions came into use.

DSM-II had a category called "anxiety neurosis," which DSM-III divided into two types. One was more chronic (GAD), characterized by constant worry and physical symptoms. The other was more acute (panic disorder, characterized by recurrent attacks). The main reason for this separation was the idea that GAD and panic depend on different pathological pathways and require different methods of treatment (Klein, 1987; Norton et al., 1995).

The clinical picture of panic disorder is one of the classic syndromes in psychiatry. Its definition has not changed in DSM-5. Generalized anxiety disorder is retained in DSM-5 but has been renamed as *"generalized anxiety and worry disorder."* This reflects a key feature: worry about events that are unlikely to happen. Other changes involve a less chronic course (excessive anxiety and worry occurring on more days than not for 3 months or longer, rather than 6 months, as in DSM-IV), a list of symptoms related more specifically to worry, a set of behaviors associated with worry, and a reduced number of required associated symptoms (1 of 4, rather than 3 of 6). These shifts may be minor, but they could greatly increase the prevalence of the disorder. Generalized anxiety disorder is defined as chronic, but reducing the time scale may dilute some distinctions. Andrews and Hobbs (2010) tested the DSM-5 proposals in community and clinical samples and did not observe increased prevalence, but this reassuring finding needs to be replicated. As we have seen, even minor changes in wording in DSM manuals can lead to diagnostic "epidemics."

Generalized anxiety disorder is not a precise diagnosis and has high levels of comorbidity with other disorders, including phobias, depression, and substance abuse (Stein, 2001). Patients with GAD or MDD have different symptom patterns (Kessler et al., 2010), so the decision to separate them was probably right. Moffitt et al. (2010), reporting on long-term follow-up studies of children who had been anxious and depressed, found that anxiety and mood problems showed longitudinal stability and remained distinct. Thus, even when symptoms overlap, endophenotypes may not.

PHOBIAS

Phobias are familiar diagnoses. Yet because the classic picture of a specific phobia need not lead to serious dysfunction, specialists in psychiatry rarely see these cases. Agoraphobia, on the other hand, is not a phobia at all but a complication of panic disorder (Wittchen et al., 2010). One change in DSM-5 is to remove the requirement that phobias be recognized by patients who suffer from them as irrational. Not all patients understand this point. But Zimmerman et al. (2010) found that making that change has little effect on diagnosis.

Social phobia (or social anxiety disorder) has attracted attention because it appears to be common (Davidson et al., 1993). However, given the high prevalence of social anxiety and shyness in community populations, this category may be too broadly defined (Wakefield et al., 2005). To give a diagnosis to anyone who has trouble speaking in public or attending a social event is another example of mission creep (not to speak of disease-mongering). And because antidepressants have been widely promoted for treatment, this diagnosis has opened a lucrative market for the pharmaceutical industry. Some have even suggested that social phobia was invented specifically to market medication to a large number of people previously considered to be normally shy (Lane, 2007).

Finally, "separation anxiety disorder" (formerly school phobia) has been moved from the childhood section to the anxiety disorders chapter. We need more research to determine how this syndrome develops and changes in adult life.

POST-TRAUMATIC STRESS DISORDER AND ACUTE STRESS DISORDER

These diagnoses are placed by DSM-5 in a separate chapter related to trauma and stress. But almost all mental disorders have some relationship to adverse life events. Moreover, disorders considered to be "post-traumatic" also reflect biological predispositions, as well as social factors that shape clinical presentation. The idea that PTSD is one of the few disorders for which we know the etiology is mistaken. Most people who are exposed to trauma don't develop PTSD, and those who do usually have past symptomatology (McNally, 2009).

Post-traumatic stress disorder was a new diagnosis in DSM-III and has been controversial since. The criteria have often been criticized (McNally, 2009), and changed in every edition of the manual. Yet clinicians love this diagnosis, probably because it suggests an etiology. Researchers understand that etiology is highly complex. But clinicians can be tempted by the simplicity of cause and effect. The DSM-5 definition combines a putative cause (a traumatic event) with a set of characteristic symptoms. Criterion A describes the trauma: an event that is either life threatening, could lead to serious injury, or rape. However, the diagnosis has been broadened by allowing incidents that consist only of hearing about trauma, which could expand the prevalence of PTSD.

Roberts et al. (2012) found that the nature of the trauma makes little difference to response, suggesting that this is a syndrome that reflects more about intrinsic sensitivity than about a reaction to life-threatening events. There are four groups of symptoms characterizing the syndrome: intrusion (re-experiencing the trauma), avoidance (avoiding situations that elicit memories), alternations in cognition and mood, as well as increased arousal. All must last for more than a month.

Using DSM-IV criteria, the community prevalence of PTSD is high: 7.8% (Kessler et al., 1995). That could suggest problems with the diagnosis. First and foremost is the Criterion A problem, as it is not clear what is meant by the word "traumatic" (Breslau & Kessler, 2001).

Is a trauma a stressor that everyone would feel deeply upset by (such as a direct threat to one's own life), or is it really enough to be a bystander or a distant observer (e.g., watching a terrorist attack on TV)? Do you have to be flooded with fear or horror at the time, as DSM-IV required? Do common experiences such as loss and grief qualify as traumas? These problems have affected the validity of research on PTSD since the diagnosis was included in DSM-III (Spitzer et al., 2007). The DSM-5 definition no longer requires people to feel "traumatized" at first expo-sure. That opens the door to attributing one's symptoms to a traumatic event retrospectively, creating an illusion of cause and effect. Specifically DSM-5 allows being a witness to disaster, or even reactions to learning about disasters, to be a traumatic event (Friedman et al., 2011). These criteria are insufficiently restrictive and may mislead clinicians to ignore intrinsic factors behind the emergence of symptoms.

A second problem concerns the use of PTSD in clinical prac-tice. Patients who report a severe trauma may receive this diagnosis, whether or not symptoms are actually related to the event. Even divorce or bereavement can sometimes be counted as "traumatic." Once one accepts the expansion of PTSD, the majority of the population could end up being "survivors." As McNally (2009) points out, overdiagno-sis weakens the concept and fails to focus on a key idea—the impact of severe trauma.

A third problem concerns the extent to which PTSD is a reaction to trauma, as opposed to the uncovering of a temperamental vulner-ability to stress. It is well established that most people exposed to trauma, even severe trauma, *never* develop PTSD (Paris, 2000). The most common response to traumatic exposure is not disorder but resil-ience and recovery. Post-traumatic stress disorder is as much a conse-quence of personality traits as of life events. For example, McFarlane (1989) showed that PTSD in firefighters was best predicted by traits of neuroticism *prior* to exposure, rather than by the severity of fires. The same conclusion has emerged in studies of PTSD in large community samples (Breslau et al., 1991).

In summary, PTSD is a syndrome marked by heterogeneity (Rosen & Lilienfeld, 2008), which is a problem for research. Some cases are pro-totypical, but as with so many other mental disorders, symptoms vary greatly from patient to patient, and there are no consistent biological markers.DSM-5 has made a few changes in the definition of PTSD but has not narrowed down the definition of a traumatic event. One can only hope that clinicians will use their common sense and not overdiagnose a condition that already suffers from inflated prevalence.

The clinical features of PTSD described in DSM-IV (hyperarousal, intrusive memories, avoidance of stimuli that re-evoke the response have been retained. The addition of a fourth dimension, alterations in cognition and mood, may be a good idea, but the inclusion of dissociative and aggressive symptoms could create a confusing overlap with personality disorders.

The major unsolved problem, as with so many other disorders in DSM-5, is the boundary with normality. Post-traumatic stress disorder is another example of how easy it is to expand a psychiatric category to the point that it describes phenomena that are not actually pathological. Life is full of adversity—it never really gives us a break. Post-traumatic stress disorder has suffered from diagnostic inflation and should be reserved for patients disabled by traumatic memories and avoidance many months after a negative life event. Prior to 1 month, these reactions constitute an "acute stress reaction," a syndrome that is much more common. The diagnosis is somewhat restricted by a time requirement, in that PTSD must meet full criteria for several months. However, there has always been and will still be a gap between describing *every* extended reaction to adversity, no matter what the clinical picture, and in the absence of characteristic symptoms, as a form of PTSD. Although one cannot blame DSM for the problem, it does little to warn clinicians about overdiagnosis. And the clinician's trap of seeing every response to trauma as PTSD only succeeds in making the concept trivial. That would be "mission creep" indeed.

There are political and historical reasons why PTSD has been defined in such a broad way. Like other categories in psychiatry, it can be used to convey social meaning. The diagnosis carries a powerful emotional punch and provides *validation* for reactions to adversity. Patients may like the diagnosis, because suffering from PTSD allows them to consider themselves as victims of circumstance. It is not an accident that the introduction of this diagnosis into the manual came at a time when large numbers of Vietnam veterans were being seen at VA hospitals, creating a need for a diagnostic concept to frame treatment (Young, 1997). But most war veterans do not develop PTSD, and those who seek treatment have other problems. Moreover, rates of disorder in the veteran population were greatly overestimated—it was even found that some claimants for benefits on the basis of this diagnosis had never been in combat (McNally, 2003). Young (1997) observed that many cases were shoe-horned into a PTSD diagnosis to justify free treatment for a very wide variety of symptoms.

In summary, DSM-5 has tinkered with PTSD but has not addressed its problems. As it stands, the diagnosis fails to consider wide individual variations in response to life events. The definition fails to correct the widely believed but oversimplified and mistaken impression that trauma is the sole or main cause of this disorder.

OBSESSIVE-COMPULSIVE DISORDER

Obsessive-compulsive disorder, and conditions in the OCD spectrum, are now in their own separate chapter. Although every psychiatrist sees patients with this diagnosis, it is far from easy to treat (Stein & Fineberg, 2007).

The definition of OCD has not changed in DSM-5. It describes a picture of obsessions and compulsions (most patients have both) that lead to significant dysfunction. The classical picture, in which patients can spend hours on rituals, is easy to diagnose, although the most severe cases present symptoms that seem uncomfortably close to psychosis.

Obsessive-compulsive disorder is believed to lie in a spectrum that includes body dysmorphic disorder, trichotillomania, stereotypic movement disorder (tics), pediatric auto-immune neuropsychiatric disorders associated with streptococcal infections (PANDAS), as well as obsessive-compulsive personality disorder (Fineberg et al., 2010). But research on these relationships is thin. For example, although family studies find that these disorders cluster together (Hollander et al., 2009), more families are seen in which spectrum disorders are *not* found than those in which they are present.

In the OCD spectrum, the decision to add a new diagnosis of "hoarding disorder" (Mataix-Cols et al., 2010) has aroused controversy. This syndrome may not qualify as a separately diagnosable mental disorder, as it describes a single symptom (previously considered a sign of obsessive-compulsive personality disorder). Media reports have sometimes described patients dying as a result of being trapped in their own hoard, but such cases are rare. Hoarding is common in attenuated forms that affect as many as 5% of the general population (Samuels et al., 2008). Obviously, quite a few people hate to throw things out. (Interest in this problem even inspired a TV "reality" program.) But to diagnose a mental disorder, patients need to be functionally disabled. The DSM-5 definition includes difficulty in parting with possessions, associated with an urge to save them, the accumulation of possessions, and clinically significant distress or functional impairment. Although it may be useful to put this problem, which all clinicians see from time to time, in the manual, it remains to be seen whether the syndrome will be better understood.

Three other conditions have made their entry into this group. Body dysmorphic disorder has been moved from somatic conditions to the OCD-related spectrum. So has hair-pulling disorder (trichotillomania). Both have common features with OCD, but no one knows why some people have obsessive thoughts and carry out rituals, whereas others worry about their appearance or pull their hair. This is uncharted territory. Finally, skin-picking (excoriation) disorder has been added to the list.

In spite of these changes, anxiety disorders have not been radically revised in DSM-5. This is fortunate, as they have not benefited from as much research as mood disorders.

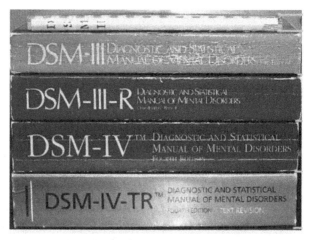

DSM manuals—how they grew larger

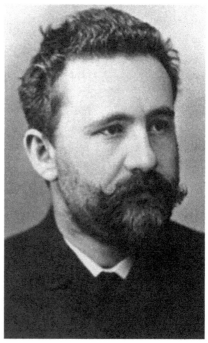

Emil Kraepelin—pioneer of diagnosis

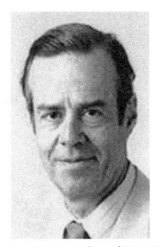

Robert Spitzer—editor of DSM-III

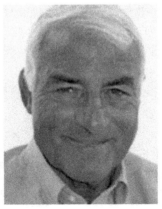

Allen Frances—editor of DSM-IV and critic of DSM-5

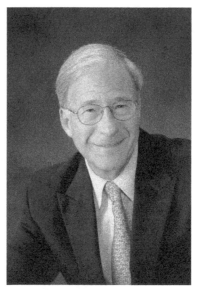

David Kupfer—co-editor of DSM-5

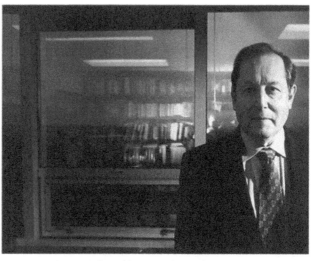

Darryl Regier—co-editor of DSM-5

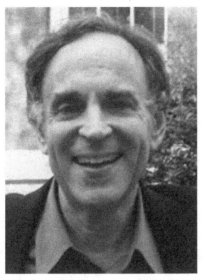

Jerome Wakefield—working to separate mental disorder from normality

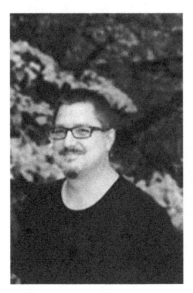

Robert Krueger—promoter of dimensionality

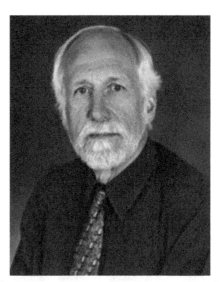

William Carpenter—promoter of attenuated psychosis

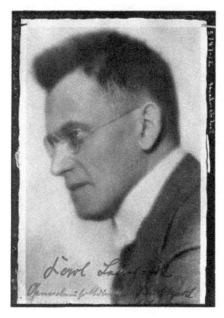

Karl Leonhardt—creator of "bipolar"

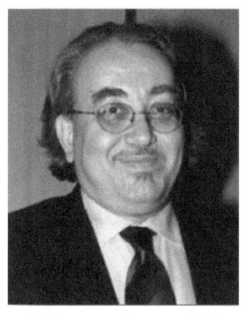

Hagop Akiskal—promoter of depressive and bipolar spectra

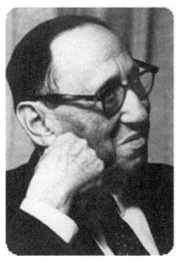

Leo Kanner—pioneer of autism

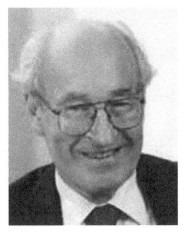

Michael Rutter—dean of child psychiatry

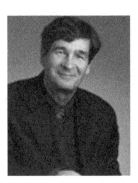

John Gunderson—dean of personality disorder research

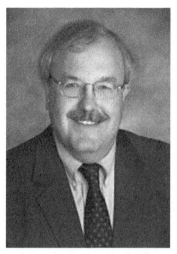

Andrew Skodol—chair of personality disorder work group

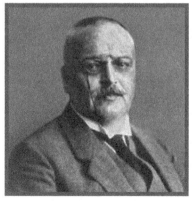

Alois Alzheimer—pioneer of dementia

Chapter 11

Substance Use, Eating, and Sexual Disorders

THE BOUNDARIES OF SUBSTANCE USE AND ADDICTION

Substance use disorder and addiction provide an instructive instance of the difficulty of establishing a boundary between normality and mental disorder. We live in a culture where most people drink alcohol, and in which excess intake from time to time is far from unusual. Since the 1960s, one could say much the same about marijuana. The chapter in DSM-5 also includes addictions to behaviors, not just to substances. The main modification is that there is no longer any categorical difference between substance use and addiction. The media have duly noted that more people will be diagnosed as having an addiction.

What determines the boundary between use and addiction? DSM, in its various editions, has focused on maladaptive patterns of use leading to "clinically significant impairment or distress." But that concept lacks a precise definition. Less sensitive criteria such as "committing illegal acts" have been removed, and a new criterion of "craving" has been added to the definition. Even so, deciding what is or is not clinically significant requires a judgment call. Does impairment depend on losing one's job and/or losing intimate relationships? Can one be sure that these outcomes would not have happened anyway? One is on safer ground in focusing on the physical effects of substance use. But those sequelae only emerge after years of use.

This boundary problem helps to explain why substance use disorders have such a high prevalence in epidemiological studies. In the ECA study, about 10% of all men in the United States met lifetime criteria for alcoholism (Robins & Regier, 1991). In the NCS-R, 13.2% met lifetime criteria for alcohol abuse, and with a further 5.4% for alcohol dependence, the total was more than 18% (Kessler et al., 2005a). Reflecting the tendency of alcoholism to remit, the National Epidemiologic Survey on Alcohol and Related Conditions (NESARC; Grant et al., 2004b) reported a 12-month prevalence for alcohol abuse of 4.7%, with 3.8% for dependence. A high lifetime prevalence of alcoholism could be a cause for alarm, given that many who abuse alcohol never seek treatment. But it is also possible that these numbers are inflated by an overly broad definition of the disorder.

SUBSTANCE USE AND ADDICTION IN DSM-5

DSM-5 defines a substance use disorder as a maladaptive pattern leading to clinically significant impairment or distress for at least 12 months. These features must meet 2 or more of the following 11 criteria: recurrent substance use leading to a failure to fulfill major role obligations, associated with social and interpersonal problems, in situations that are physically hazardous, tolerance (need for increased amounts or diminished effect of the same amount), withdrawal effects, taking the substance in larger amounts and for longer than intended, unsuccessful efforts at cutting down, spending time to obtain or use the substance, giving up other activities, continuing despite the problem, and craving the substance. A criterion has been added: "Craving or a strong desire or urge to use a specific substance." A previous criterion describing legal problems has been dropped (as not predictive of dysfunction). There are severity specifiers, depending on the number of criteria met (greater than 4 is considered severe). DSM-5 also describes course specifiers (early full remission, early partial remission, sustained full remission, sustained partial remission on agonist therapy in a controlled environment).

Each drug follows the same general guideline. Clinicians are also asked to specify whether physiological dependence is present. Note that the term "dependence" is reserved for tolerance and/or withdrawal symptoms. This definition is broad and dimensional, but many patients can be diagnosed if they meet only two criteria. Martin et al. (2011) criticized this requirement as too lenient. Yet it goes along with the manual's overall philosophy, which is to include subclinical phenomena within a spectrum.

The chair of the work group (O'Brien, 2011) has defended these changes. "Dependence" was eliminated because it is a confusing concept that conflates physical and psychological need for a substance. The logic depends on research suggesting that alcoholism is dimensional (Hasin & Beseler, 2009). Thus, a disorder can be rated on a continuum of severity and then coded for physiological dependence. Thus addiction will be identified by a dimensional scoring procedure based on severity (Shields et al., 2007).

In the past, the term "addiction" always required physiological dependence. It might increase stigma to use this term for binge drinkers and for anyone else who misuses alcohol. Once again, seeing pathology on a continuum runs the danger of watering down diagnostic concepts. Basing diagnosis on severity also masks the fact that different clinical presentations may require different treatment.

The question is whether DSM-5 will make these diagnoses more frequent. An Australian survey (Mewton et al., 2011) found that using the DSM-5 criteria could lead to a 60% increase in prevalence in substance use disorders as a whole. An American study (Agrawal et al., 2011) found only a 10% increase. Either way, this would be a significant change.

This brings us back to the same basic problem: the absence of a clear boundary between using too much and having an addiction problem. Everything depends on assessment of impairment. At what point is a patient who drinks to excess failing to meet major role obligations? In severe cases, the answer is obvious. In the more common and milder cases, it may not be.

BEHAVIORAL ADDICTIONS

DSM applies the same concepts to "behavioral addictions." Pathological gambling is an example. In the NCS-R (Kessler et al., 2008), this diagnosis had a lifetime prevalence of 0.6%, although it was highly comorbid with other disorders.

Gambling problems have a similar form and function to substance abuse. There is an attraction to addictive behavior, resulting in failure to perform major role obligations, as well as continuance despite negative consequences. DSM-5 has therefore moved "disordered gambling" from the DSM-IV group of impulse disorders to the substance group. But other addictive behaviors are still classified elsewhere. Bulimia nervosa also resembles an addiction, in that the process of binging and purging can provide quick relief from dysphoric emotions (Brisman & Siegel, 1984). Another example is self-harm, common in borderline personality disorder, which can be addictive because it provides immediate relief for dysphoric emotions (Linehan, 1993).

Internet addiction, a more recent phenomenon, is not included in DSM-5. Research has described people who give up all other activities to be (or to live) online (Block, 2008). But caution is needed, as one would have to define a boundary between addiction and the difficulty many people have in ending sessions on the Internet. We also do not know whether this problem is a reflection of other mental disorders or a disorder in its own right.

The development of new addictive behaviors can be explained by Shorter's (1993) concept of a "symptom pool." Many symptoms in psychiatry are socially and historically determined. Each era provides a particular venue, technological or otherwise, for the expression of distress. The danger is that seeing too wide range of symptoms in an addiction model tries to account for too much, but explains too little.

ANOREXIA NERVOSA

The next chapter of DSM-5 describes Feeding and Eating Disorders. Anorexia nervosa has been recognized as a mental disorder since the early nineteenth century (Shorter, 1993). Its characteristic feature is a weight loss of at least 15% below standard norms, accompanied by a pursuit of thinness (Grilo & Mitchell, 2010). Anorexics have an abnormal body image and can see themselves as overweight even when their life is in danger. Mortality is high, with more than 5% dying per decade after diagnosis, either from physical complications or suicide (Sullivan, 1995). The clinical picture can be further divided into a restricting type (reduced intake and high levels of exercise) and a purging type (also involving bulimic episodes and use of laxatives to reduce weight).

There is little doubt that anorexia nervosa qualifies as a distinct illness. However, it reflects a strong cultural factor, the preference of modern society for thin women (Garner & Garfinkel, 1980). The syndrome is unknown in cultures where food is scarce and famine possible and only begins to appear in developed societies such as North America and Western Europe—only when food is ubiquitous does one see cultural preferences for a slim body (Brumberg, 1988).

The boundary between over-concern about body image and anorexia nervosa is porous. A community survey found that anorexia itself, mainly seen in young females, affected nearly 1% of women (Hudson et al., 2007). That figure is high, and may reflect too broad a definition. We should be careful to distinguish between the classical syndrome (which is life-threatening) and less severe variants.

The DSM-5 definition is similar to past editions: restriction of intake associated with serious weight loss, fear of gaining weight, and a body image disturbance. One is asked to specify a subtype—restricting or binge-eating/purging. Some changes have been introduced into DSM-5: refusal to eat and fear of weight gain are replaced by focusing on behaviors that keep weight low. The most substantive change is the deletion of a requirement for amenorrhea, which, as shown years ago (Garfinkel et al., 1996), may or may not be present. These minor changes should not make it more difficult to recognize anorexia nervosa.

BULIMIA NERVOSA

The other major eating disorder, bulimia nervosa, is characterized by binge-eating, a loss of control, and compensatory behavior such as purging, at least twice a week for 3 months. Bulimia affects 1.5% of women in the general population (Hudson et al., 2007). It can be distinguished from binge-eating, which has a much higher prevalence (3.5% of women), and from the "experimental" purging seen in some normal adolescents. Bulimia nervosa is an excellent example of how culture shapes psychopathology. It was described only a few decades ago by the British psychiatrist Gerald Russell (1979). I cannot remember seeing a single case during my residency 40 years ago. Today it is a social epidemic.

DSM-5 has made few changes in the definition. The most substantive is that episodes of binge-eating can now occur once a week over 3 months, as opposed to twice a week in DSM-IV. Although there is no empirically determined boundary for frequency, as with other diagnoses in DSM-5, the revision leans toward including subclinical cases.

BINGE-EATING DISORDER

Binge-eating disorder (BED) is a diagnosis that has aroused controversy. It is a new category, moved up from the Appendix of DSM-IV. Binge-eating disorder was by far the most prevalent eating disorder in the National Comorbidity Survey Replication (Hudson et al., 2007). Severe binging would previously have been covered by the DSM-IV category of eating disorder NOS, which had been introduced to describe patients who did not meet criteria for anorexia or bulimia. Some research has suggested that eating disorders lie on a continuum, with BED being a less severe form (Wonderlich et al., 2009).

The diagnosis describes recurrent episodes of binge-eating (on average, at least once a week for 3 months, eating a large amount of food in a short time, and a sense of lack of control over eating during the episode). Episodes must also be associated with three (or more) of the following: eating much more rapidly than normal, eating until uncomfortably full, eating large amounts of food when not physically hungry, eating alone, feeling disgusted with oneself, marked distress. But binge-eating is not associated with the recurrent use of inappropriate compensatory behavior (i.e., purging).

Binge-eating disorder is controversial for the same reason as most of the innovations in DSM-5. It describes symptoms that are fairly common and that may or may not deserve to be classified as mental disorders. Like sadness, occasional binge-eating is something many (if not most) of us can relate to. But does a behavior, however distressing, that occurs only a few times a month belong in a diagnostic manual? We do not diagnose alcoholism so liberally. Frances (2010a) has recommended that eating disorders be restricted to the classical forms that are known to produce severe dysfunction. Binge-eating disorder might have been omitted, or at least defined more narrowly.

Finally, this chapter of DSM-5 includes feeding disorders in early childhood. Perhaps there was no better place to put them. But "avoidant/restrictive food intake disorder" (Bryant-Waugh et al., 2010) lacks an empirical literature, seems mainly to describe picky eaters, and may only encourage parents who already worry too much about how their children are eating to be even more concerned.

In a commentary on the DSM-5 changes, Fairburn (2011) has noted that the most common form of eating disorder has been "NOS," suggesting either a failure of the system to classify cases that lie outside a few prototypes or an overextension of the eating disorder concept. A study comparing DSM-IV and DSM-5 criteria in a community sample (Keel et al., 2011) showed that diagnoses in the NOS category are reduced by DSM-5, largely because of the introduction of BED. If eating disorders will be diagnosed more frequently under the new system, this could be still one more example of how DSM confuses illness with normal variation.

SEXUAL DYSFUNCTIONS, GENDER DYSPHORIA, AND PARAPHILIAS

The next three chapters of DSM-5 concern sexual disorders (sexual dysfunctions, gender dysphoria, and paraphilias), all of which, like sex itself, have long been a subject of controversy. It is difficult to make coherent groupings, but one way to justify a separation is that dysfunctions in sexual arousal or performance are distressing, so that patients tend to come for help. People with paraphilias may be satisfied with the way they are, but patients with gender dysphoria may seek sex-change surgery.

Some sexual problems lie close to the borders of normal variation. Should psychiatrists consider them mental disorders? There is always a danger that diagnoses could oppress people who are different but not ill. There is also a danger in using diagnosis to justify treatment that is not curative but cosmetic. When it comes to sex, it is difficult to say what is normal and what is not. Nor is it clear that the medicalization of sexual difficulties yields diagnoses that have the same validity as other disorders.

Sexual Dysfunctions: These diagnoses include erectile disorder and female orgasmic disorder. DSM-5 also has categories for delayed ejaculation, early ejaculation, and disorders or sexual interest or arousal. Psychiatrists rarely treat such conditions but may be asked to consult about them and/or to make a differential diagnosis. The criteria were not changed from DSM-IV.

A new category proposed for this section, which the media found amusing, ended up in the Appendix: *hypersexual disorder.* That diagnosis would require that over a period of at least 6 months, recurrent and intense sexual fantasies, sexual urges, and sexual behavior in association with four or more of the following: excessive time consumed by sexual fantasies and urges, repetitively engaging in sexual fantasies and behavior in response to dysphoric mood states, doing the same in response to stressful life events, unsuccessful efforts to control or significantly reduce sexual fantasies and behavior, or engaging in sexual behavior while disregarding the risk for harm to self or others. In addition diagnosis requires clinically significant personal distress and/or impairment in social, occupational, or other important areas of functioning. Kafka (2010) has supported hypersexuality as an addiction, but not much is known about why some are hypersexual or why others are hyposexual. This diagnosis seems to be yet another invasion of the realm of normal variation. Once we start down that road, we might as well start diagnosing body-builders and bookworms—or almost any other behavioral pattern that differs noticeably from the norm.

Gender Dysphoria: A diagnosis of gender dysphoria describes people who, since childhood, have wanted to belong to the opposite sex (Zucker, 2010). DSM-5 defines it as incongruence between experienced gender and secondary sex characteristics, with a desire to be rid of these characteristics and to be the other gender. Cases usually first present in adolescence (Manners, 2009).

In the past, if someone experienced this kind of problem, then there was nothing to be done about it, other than cross-dressing. However, after 1950, it became possible to undergo surgery and to take on the identity of a transsexual (now called "transgendered"). Since then, psychiatrists have seen more cases fitting the clinical picture. Social contagion has increased the prevalence of the condition. Patients can learn to say what is necessary to get hormonal and/or surgical treatment (e.g., "I have always felt like a woman in a man's body.").

The gay and lesbian communities have defended the validity of a transsexual identity, describing themselves as part of a "LGBT" coalition (lesbians, gays, bisexuals, and transsexuals). In that view, gender identity disorder, like homosexuality, should *not* be a mental disorder. Of course, physicians could still treat people who are not sick, as plastic surgeons do. Usually, transsexuals are usually managed first with hormones, and only then with surgery.

Paul McHugh, Chair of Psychiatry at Johns Hopkins for many years, strongly opposed any surgical option and banned it at his hospital. McHugh (2005) argued that if no physician would remove a normal organ or body part simply on request (as opposed to requests for shaping), then they should not do so for intact genitalia. To carry out such a procedure, one would have to be convinced that a wish to have the body of the opposite sex is the product of a biological anomaly. No one has shown that to be the case.

Also, although patients with gender identity disorder claim to have *always* felt that way since childhood, no prospective follow-up studies of children have confirmed whether this is true. Reported memories may reflect more about the present than the past. A classic study of boys who preferred to play with dolls and cross-dress found that most became homosexual, rather than transsexual (Green, 1987).

Kenneth Zucker, the psychologist who chaired the sexual disorders task force for DSM-5, has studied gender identity problems in children (Zucker & Bradley, 1995), and the argument for reversing it depends on negative consequences in childhood (Cohen-Kettenis et al., 2003). But there is no evidence that that is possible. Zucker, as well as his colleague Ray Blanchard (2005), came under attack early in the DSM-5 process from activists in the LGBT community who feared that a diagnosis would be used to invalidate gender dysphoria. The driving force behind this dispute was politics, not science. In the end, DSM-5 did not change its criteria.

Paraphilias: This is the most controversial grouping among sexual disorders. The historical context is that DSM-I and DSM-II classified homosexuality as a mental disorder. Hardly anyone disagreed with doing so when I was a student, although it was widely understood that changing sexual orientation was impractical or impossible. Gradually, the view that homosexuality is a normal variant gained ground. After the 1970 APA meeting in San Francisco was interrupted by protests from the gay community, the category was removed in 1973 by a vote of the APA (Spitzer, 1981). DSM-III retained a diagnosis of "ego-dystonic homosexuality," reserved for those not happy with their sexual orientation. In DSM-IV, even that compromise was eliminated, although it remained possible to diagnose a grab-bag category of "sexual disorder, not otherwise specified." Spitzer, despite his support for homosexuals, came under attack from activists for describing cases in which a few patients switched to heterosexuality (Spitzer, 2003), and in 2012, he apologized for publishing this paper.

The controversy about homosexuality is a paradigmatic example of how diagnosis is influenced by cultural and social beliefs. Almost everyone today agrees that diagnosing same-sex attraction as a mental disorder was a mistake. But that is only one example among many in which normal variations are seen as pathology. One wishes that DSM had learned more from the homosexuality story and took seriously the principle that variability does not necessarily imply pathology. But people who are moody, nervous, or shy don't start advocacy groups to protect themselves from organized psychiatry.

At the same time, the success of activists in getting psychiatry to change its mind about the existence of *any* diagnosis is worrying. However justified in the case of homosexuality, the decision set a precedent. If APA can be convinced to normalize one type of sexual variation, then why should it not do so for all the others? Up to now, no one has seriously contemplated declaring pedophilia to be a normal variant. The obvious reason is that it is a crime, with victims who cannot consent. The same principle applies to exhibitionism. Yet fetishism, which hurts no one, remains in DSM-5. Frances (2010a) recommends that unusual sexual fantasies that affect no one but the person experiencing them should never be considered as mental disorders. DSM-5 fails to distinguish between paraphilias that present a social danger to other people and those that cause personal distress.

The proposed diagnosis of coercive paraphilia (Knight, 2010)—that is, rape actions or fantasies—ended up in the Appendix of the manual. This concept had problems related to diagnostic inflation. No one disagrees that rape is a crime that should be punished. But it has never previously been considered as a mental disorder, except perhaps by those who consider all crimes to be a sign of illness. The proposed criteria included wanting to rape and then either being distressed by such a fantasy or acting on it (at least three times). It is hard to see why *thinking* about doing something criminal should constitute a mental disorder. Frances (2010a) has expressed concern that this diagnosis could expand the pool of sex offenders eligible for indefinite civil commitment. All these critiques have led to putting the category in the Appendix, where it should stay.

Otherwise, there are no major changes in the classification. Pedophilic disorder has been tweaked a bit to reflect biological developmental indicators of early puberty in victims, avoiding an implication that the disorder must always involves post-pubertal adolescents.

The problems in defining sexual disorders have not been resolved by DSM-5. Some reflect theoretical confusion, some a lack of research, and some politics. These are scientific issues that cannot be resolved without more empirical data.

Chapter 12

Neurodevelopmental and Disruptive Behavioral Disorders

NEURODEVELOPMENTAL DISORDERS

These conditions have a basis in abnormal brain development early in life. The grouping includes intellectual developmental disorder (formerly called mental retardation), language developmental disorders, learning disorders, and motor disorders. In DSM-5, intellectual developmental disorder no longer categorizes patients strictly on the basis of IQ but requires a score that falls approximately two standard deviations from the mean (i.e., 70 or less).

Communication disorders, including language and speech disorders (language impairment, late language emergence, specific language impairment, and social communication impairment) are a separate grouping. Learning disorders are defined as independent of general intelligence and require confirmation with a standardized and psychometrically sound instrument. If clinicians were to follow these directives, then one might expect less of a tendency to diagnose every struggling student with a learning disorder. However, because everyone scores differently on psychological tests, these instruments could be used in the service of diagnostic inflation. Finally, motor disorders include Tourette's syndrome, a diagnosis that has attracted a fair amount of research interest.

PERVASIVE DEVELOPMENTAL (AUTISTIC SPECTRUM) DISORDERS

The American child psychiatrist Leo Kanner was the first physician to describe autism (Kanner, 1943). Illness begins before age 3 years and severely reduces social and cognitive functioning. It says something about the nature of post-war American psychiatry that autism was at first thought to be psychogenic and that mothers were blamed for its development. It took years to establish that autism was heritable and associated with functional brain abnormalities (McGregor et al., 2008).

The best-studied variant of autism is Asperger's syndrome. In 1944, the Austrian pediatrician Hans Asperger described children with poor social functioning and stereotyped behaviors (Szatmari, 2004). In DSM-IV, the syndrome was separate but fell under the broader category of *pervasive developmental disorders*. In DSM-5, both classical autism and Asperger's are folded into an autistic spectrum. That decision aroused controversy, as Asperger's does not carry the same stigma as autism.

In DSM-5, an autism spectrum disorder is defined as persistent deficits in social communication and social interaction, associated with restricted, repetitive patterns of behavior, interests, or activities. Symptoms have to begin in childhood and severely limit functioning. Previous diagnoses of childhood disintegrative disorder, and pervasive developmental disorder (not otherwise specified) are also included in the spectrum. Although some were concerned that the DSM-5 definition could be more restrictive than in DSM-IV, this does not seem to be the case (Huerta et al., 2012).

Autistic spectrum disorders suffer from most of the same problems as many other diagnostic groups. On the severe end, mental disorder is definite. On the milder end, one finds a fuzzy boundary with normal levels of introversion. The same pattern we saw for other disorders repeats itself here, with rapidly increasing diagnosis of autism by physicians (Kogan et al., 2009). This trend might be attributed to better recognition but is more likely to reflect the pathologizing of subclinical symptoms. Asperger's syndrome has become a diagnostic fad that is being applied to all kinds of "nerdy" people. Needless to say, we have no biological markers to confirm the diagnosis. Of course, DSM-5 has not hesitated to expand the boundaries of the autistic spectrum.

The result of these changes in diagnostic practice is that autism has changed from a rare disease to a very common one. A recent report from South Korea (Kim et al., 2011) got media attention by estimating the community prevalence of the autism spectrum to be 2.6%, several times higher than previous estimates (Fombonne, 2009). It has since been contradicted by a survey from the United Kingdom, which found only 1% (Brugha et al., 2011), although that is still high. All these estimates are inflated by including subclinical cases, as has been the case with the prevalence for so many disorders.

These days, all kinds of eccentric people can be labeled as having a variant of autism. Even historical figures, like Albert Einstein, are not immune from diagnosis. (Einstein may have been eccentric and nerdy, but he was not in any way autistic.) Once more, an important diagnostic concept is watered down by over-inclusion. Moreover, we do not know what causes autism, whether it reflects one or many diseases, or whether extending its boundaries will turn out to be clinically useful.

The DSM-5 definition, although hardly narrow, is more restrictive than patient activists would have wanted since it makes some attempt to counter the tendency for an "epidemic" of autism. Frazier et al. (2012) compared the new system to DSM-IV-TR and suggested relaxing requirements to include the 12% of patients (including many females) who would no longer meet criteria. Instead, DSM-5 offers a new category called "social communication disorder" that describes milder symptoms, in which verbal and nonverbal communication are impaired, without fulfilling criteria for the autism spectrum.

The New York Times (Jan 20, 2011) quoted Yale psychiatrist Fred Volkmar (a member of the autism study group) as favoring more emphasis on classical autism to avoid over-identification. Opposition to these recommendations has been political, because families of patients who would qualify for a diagnosis under broader rules are worried it could interfere with payment for expensive treatment or special schooling. This demonstrates, once again, that DSM-5 has many constituents, not all of whom are satisfied by diagnostic conservatism.

ATTENTION DEFICIT HYPERACTIVITY DISORDER

Attention deficit hyperactivity disorder (ADHD) begins, by definition, in childhood. Its prevalence in children is high: 5% in the United States, with some estimates approaching 10% in boys (Faraone et al., 2000). Prevalence is lower in other countries, and it is hard to credit any conclusion that ADHD is more common in American children. More likely, clinicians in the United States have a lower threshold for identifying the disorder. Many children are overly excited and distractible at times. At what point do these states become a mental disorder? Or do the criteria turn normal variability into a form of pathology, as one might suspect from high estimates of prevalence?

The symptoms on which clinicians base a diagnosis of ADHD in childhood are not strikingly different from past editions of DSM. A series of characteristic features are described, of which at least six are required to be present over at least 6 months. There are two subtypes, characterized by inattention or by hyperactivity and impulsivity (with the additional possibility of a mixed picture). These features must appear by age 12 years and reduce functioning. The most important revision is a later age of onset. That will definitely expand the diagnosis, as it allows for cases in which symptoms only begin on the cusp of adolescence (Batstra & Frances, 2012). Considering the likelihood that ADHD is already being overdiagnosed, this is a worrying development.

When I was a resident, in the days of DSM-II, this clinical picture was called either "hyperkinetic reaction of childhood" or "minimal brain dysfunction." But these terms were based on etiological assumptions not supported by data. DSM-III, which based diagnoses on signs and symptoms rather than on theories, therefore changed the name to Attention-Deficit Disorder (with or without hyperactivity). The current terminology, in which both features are acknowledged in the name "ADHD," was introduced in DSM-III-R. One can now diagnose children with a predominantly inattentive picture, a predominantly hyperactive picture, or a combination of both. As we will see, it is the inattentive group that arouses the most controversy.

One reason why the diagnosis of ADHD has been so popular is that it is widely believed to lead to a specific and effective method of treatment. As with bipolar disorder, psychiatrists and family doctors are attracted to any diagnosis that leads to a definite plan of action, particularly a prescription. Stimulants such as methylphenidate have been been used successfully for decades to treat hyperactive children. However, as the definition of the disorder broadened, pharmacological therapy became less specific. By and large, hyperactive symptoms respond best to medication, inattentive symptoms much less so (Leung & Lemay, 2003). This raises the question as to whether they are part of the same disorder.

It was long believed that one could confirm a diagnosis of ADHD by observing a paradoxical response to stimulants, which would calm a hyperactive child (as opposed to a stimulating effect in normal children). But these effects are not consistent. In the fuzzier domain of inattention and low concentration, stimulants may yield much the same results (increased attention and focus) in normal children as in children with ADHD (Rapoport et al., 1978).

Attention-deficit hyperactivity disorder, like so many other mental disorders, is a syndrome. It shows extensive comorbidity with other disruptive behavioral disorders of childhood, particularly conduct disorder and oppositional defiant disorder (McGee et al., 2000). These behavioral problems are more likely than ADHD itself to bring children to clinical attention. Another problem lies with the inattentive type, somewhat more common in girls, and difficult to distinguish from other causes of poor attention.

There is little doubt the diagnosis of ADHD, in typical cases and where hyperactivity is present, identifies a cohort of children in which most will respond to treatment with stimulants. The problem is whether current criteria describe too heterogeneous a population and whether some cases at the fringes might better be described (and treated) in other ways.

In recent decades there has been great interest in diagnosing ADHD in adulthood. It has long been known that childhood symptoms do not always disappear with maturity (Weiss & Hechtman, 1993). However, the boundaries of the adult syndrome are fuzzy. Moreover, clinicians need to establish that ADHD began in childhood. That simple requirement is often ignored. I have often seen the diagnosis made in people who *never* had symptoms as children. But establishing a childhood history is not easy. Clinicians must ask patients to accurately remember behavioral problems from decades ago. Moreover, some patients, convinced by the media (or their friends and family) that they must have ADHD, retell their life story in light of a preconceived conclusion. This often happens when a child is treated for the disorder, and a parent comes to the conclusion that they have the same problem. That is why clinicians should ask for school records and interview parents before making a diagnosis.

Using DSM-IV-TR criteria, the National Comorbidity Survey found a community prevalence of 4.4% for adult ADHD (Kessler et al., 2006). That is an enormous prevalence for a disorder rarely diagnosed only 20 years ago. So we have to ask whether the current DSM criteria are picking up something that clinicians have long missed or whether they are over-identifying the disorder.

Adult ADHD is highly comorbid with mood disorders, substance abuse, and personality disorders (Cumyn et al., 2009). All of these conditions can cause attention problems in their own right. There is no specific way to establish a diagnosis of ADHD independent of these comorbidities. Sometimes clinicians are left with the option of prescribing a stimulant just to see if it works. My experience is that many patients are being diagnosed with checklists such as the Conners scales (Conners & Lett, 1999), or by psychological testing, and then given stimulants. Even then, clinicians can hardly be sure that a response proves anything about the nature of the underlying psychopathology. If normal people have better attention on these drugs, and if placebo effects are powerful, it is impossible to tell.

DSM-5 has made it easier to make an ADHD diagnosis in adults. Patients now only have to demonstrate an onset prior to age 12 years (rather than 7 years) and to have three (rather than six) of the characteristic symptoms during childhood. But how one can be sure of the accuracy of a childhood history? We can expect to see a further expansion of the current "epidemic" of adult ADHD, leading to an even higher frequency of pharmacological treatment. Clinicians today often see many patients who ask for stimulants, usually based on media reports of their efficacy. DSM-5 makes it more likely that drugs will be prescribed to people who do not need them.

Adult ADHD still has to begin in childhood. But why were the criteria for age of onset extended to age 12 years? This decision was justified by community surveys that failed to show that a later onset makes any difference in course (Kieling et al., 2010; Polanczyk et al., 2010). But that assumes you can be *sure* a child has ADHD, which is impossible (without biomarkers that remain to be discovered). Being distractable or not paying attention can have many other causes, particularly when the problem does not begin in early or middle childhood, and there is an important sociocultural component to attention (Frances, 2010a). For most of human history, children worked alongside adults and were never expected to sit quietly in classrooms for hours at a time. Because most adults in the past carried out manual labor rather than desk jobs, attention was less of an issue. Attention-deficit hyperactivity disorder may be a temperamental variant that has become a serious problem in relation to the demands of modern society.

Frances (2010a) wryly notes that he holds himself responsible for the vast expansion of this diagnosis after the publication of DSM-IV. The introduction of adult ADHD, with broad criteria, led to great diagnostic inflation. This was only one example of a much larger problem. Every work group wants to expand the boundaries of the condition they study. When the manual lowers the bar, prevalence usually goes up sharply.

Giving long-term stimulant medication to millions of children has stimulated controversy. Some criticism is uninformed, as treatment is clearly effective in classical cases. But everything depends on the validity and range of the diagnosis. Fortunately, the long-term effects of stimulants are much less serious than those of antipsychotics, a group for which prescriptions in preschool children have also increased (Olfson et al., 2010). The question concerns how to distinguish children (and adults) who are most likely to benefit from stimulant treatment from those who are not (and who may need another kind of therapy). If both children and adults with ADHD are highly comorbid for other disorders, then what is primary and what is secondary? To address these dilemmas we need biological markers. And once again, that is just what we don't have.

DISRUPTIVE, IMPULSE CONTROL, AND CONDUCT DISORDERS

Disruptive behavioral disorders are the most common problems seen by child psychiatrists, In addition to ADHD, two diagnoses describe most of these cases. The milder form is oppositional defiant disorder (ODD), and the more severe form is conduct disorder (CD).

No changes have been made in the diagnosis of CD, which lists 15 symptoms and requires that 3 of them be present for at least a year. But there is an additional specifier for callous and unemotional traits, which consistently predict an outcome of antisocial personality disorder in adulthood. The problem is the polythetic definition of CD. A long list of symptoms (unchanged in DSM-5) is required for a diagnosis. A pattern of aggression to people or animals, property destruction, deceitfulness, and serious failure to follow rules is clearly pathological. But only 3 of 15 criteria are required for the diagnosis, making CD one of the most heterogeneous diagnoses in a manual replete with heterogeneity. Only some of this variation is captured by the severity modifiers in DSM-5 (mild, moderate, or severe).

Pardini et al. (2010) summarized the issues that require further research: whether the existing criteria work for girls, whether requiring the presence of callous–unemotional traits defines a valid subtype, and whether dimensional conceptualizations of ODD and CD can be justified. By and large, ODD and CD are broad diagnoses that describe a range of behavioral problems. As with depression, disorders that cover too a wide range may eventually need to be divided up. But that cannot happen until we have a better knowledge of causes.

Conduct disorder is worrisome because up to half of children with this diagnosis develop psychopathy and/or antisocial personality disorder in adulthood. This relationship was established decades ago, in a study of children seen in psychiatry followed up longitudinally for several decades (Robins, 1966). Later, it was shown that the most severe cases with an early onset (before age 3 years) are most likely to have an antisocial outcome, that callous and unemotional traits increase the risk, and that less severe symptoms are more likely to be precursors of mood and anxiety disorders (Zocolillo et al., 1992). The later CD starts, the better the prognosis: Cases with an onset during adolescence usually recover by young adulthood (Moffitt et al., 1993). These teenagers are influenced by peer groups, and most grow up to regret their youthful follies.

Oppositional defiant disorder also requires only four of eight listed symptoms, characterized by negativistic, hostile, and defiant behaviors that interfere with functioning. Although some cases of ODD eventually meet criteria for conduct disorder (Loeber et al., 2000), symptoms tend to disappear with age (Maughan et al., 2004). Transitions from ODD to CD may not be frequent enough to consider them as part of the same spectrum (Rowe et al., 2010; Burke et al., 2010). Moreover, the boundaries of ODD remain problematic. Many children have oppositional behaviors, and almost every child shows them some of the time. The pattern has to be present in multiple situations (not just with teachers or parents), and a requirement has been added that children be oppositional most of the time. In the end, one still has to decide on clinical grounds whether to diagnose ODD.

Because disruptive behavioral disorders can present with mood instability, and some of the most severe cases of this kind may be diagnosed as pediatric bipolar disorder. However, members of the DSM-5 task force were cautious about the concept of bipolar disorder in pre-pubertal children, in part because it leads to frequent prescriptions of mood stabilizers and antipsychotics (Olfson et al., 2006).

DSM-5 has therefore introduced a new term, focusing on children who are more likely to be angry and irritable than sad or "high." That is the genesis of the introduction of a new category, *disruptive mood dysregulation disorder*, a condition mainly defined by frequent outbursts of rage in children older than age 6 years. There is little research to back up this new category, which is, puzzlingly, listed under depressive disorders rather than under disruptive behavior disorders. In any case, because children often have temper tantrums, and usually grow out of them, one should be careful about giving a psychiatric diagnosis. Doing so is discouraged by requiring that children be at least 6 years old. Even so, it is not clear whether this diagnosis will discourage aggressive pharmacological treatment in children associated with diagnoses of pediatric bipolar disorder.

IMPULSE-CONTROL DISORDERS NOT ELSEWHERE CLASSIFIED

This group is an "orphan" left over from previous manuals that does not find a place anywhere else. (Sometimes diagnoses that don't fit actually end up getting separate chapters.) But this group includes two important conditions that psychiatrists often see. One, pathological gambling, has been moved to the group of addictions. A second category, intermittent explosive disorder (IED), describes uncontrolled episodes of rage. Thus, IED does for anger what GAD does for anxiety and what dysthymia does for sadness. (When any emotion is out of control, DSM tends to convert that into a disorder.)

The empirical literature on IED is thin. An epidemiological study (Kessler et al., 2008) suggested that IED is common in the community, with a lifetime prevalence of 7% and a 12-month prevalence of 4%. These are high numbers. But given the imprecise criteria for the diagnosis, I wonder if researchers counted everyone with "road rage" as a case. Similar questions arise concerning a recent report claiming that IED can be diagnosed in 7.8% of all adolescents (McLaughlin et al., 2012). Once again, epidemiology is suspect when it relies on fuzzy DSM definitions. The main proponent of this diagnosis, Emil Coccaro (2010), a professor at the University of Chicago, has argued that IED is caused by abnormal serotonin activity. The diagnosis has sometimes been used in court to reduce assault charges (when actions were unplanned or impulsive). In DSM-5, no revision has been recommended. But the jury is out on the validity of this diagnosis.

Chapter 13

Personality Disorders

Personality disorder (PD) is my subspecialty. But that is not the reason why this chapter will cover this group of disorders in somewhat greater detail. DSM-5 had proposed more radical changes than for any other diagnostic grouping. They were a leading edge in a long-term plan to dimensionalize all diagnoses in psychiatry. But these proposals were much too difficult for clinicians to master and understand. In December, 2012, they were rejected on scientific grounds. Because there was no time to start over, the DSM-IV system was reinstated. This must be counted as the most dramatic retreat for the agenda of DSM-5.

A BRIEF HISTORY OF PERSONALITY
DISORDER DIAGNOSES

Personality disorders have been the subject of a very large research literature, most of it published in recent decades. The essential element of a PD is that it is not an *episodic* condition in an otherwise well-functioning individual. Rather, it is a chronic dysfunction that begins early in life and is slow to change.

Some diagnoses of personality disorder were associated with psychoanalysis. That is ironic, because Freud never accepted the concept, seeing most symptoms as "neurotic." But as psychoanalysts changed their goals from the removal of symptoms to personality change, the construct entered the analytic literature. The first description of pathological personality was published in the 1930s (Reich, 1933/1949), but PD only became a subject of empirical research in the 1970s and 1980s. Thus PD research has a shorter tradition than schizophrenia or bipolar

disorder (Berrios, 1993). People with these problems were not traditionally recognized as mentally disordered but as having a "bad character."
Even today, the concept of personality disorder can sometimes be dismissed as applicable only to the "worried well"—that is, an idea that
only Woody Allen would take seriously. Yet research shows that these
patients can be as dysfunctional as those with severe mood disorders
(Skodol et al., 2005).

WHY PERSONALITY DISORDERS ARE IGNORED

Personality disorder, long neglected and misunderstood, is the
Cinderella of psychiatric diagnosis. One reason is that patients with
these problems are not always likeable. They can be seen as difficult
rather than sick and may be rejected, with problems dismissed. Even so,
cases do not go away when ignored. Personality disorder is very common in psychiatric clinics, accounting for up to one-fourth of all cases
(Zimmerman et al., 2005). Unless a diagnosis is made, patients will not
receive helpful treatment. Moreover, PD patients are often misdiag-
nosed, usually with depression or bipolarity. This is a particular problem
in borderline personality. Zimmerman and Mattia (1999b) have shown
that borderline personality disorder (BPD) is frequently missed, which
leads to bad treatment. When any PD is comorbid with depression, treatment of mood symptoms alone tends to be ineffective (Newton-Howes
et al., 2006). The presence of a personality disorder also makes it much
more likely that depression will recur (Skodol et al., 2011). And because
some patients have a highly unstable mood, there is a high frequency of
misdiagnosis of bipolar disorder, leading to unnecessary and harmful
drug treatment.

How did this problem arise? First, PDs have been defined and
described in ways that do not always make sense to clinicians. The concept is complex, particularly in comparison to mood disorder. Second, it
is difficult to separate personality (which we all have) from personality
disorder (which only some have). Again, the boundary between normality and pathology is not clear. Third, PDs do not respond well to medication and are more effectively treated with psychotherapy (Paris, 2008c).

Because that conclusion does not fit the current zeitgeist of psychiatry, attempts have been made to redefine the clinical problem by using diagnoses that justify pharmacotherapy. Finally, it is not just a prejudice that PD patients can be troublesome. Some are very difficult indeed.

The overall concept of a PD is not easy to grasp. The first formal definition, which appeared in DSM-IV, stated that PD describes an enduring, inflexible, and pervasive pattern of inner experience and behavior that begins in late adolescence or early adulthood and that continues to impede functioning in work and relationships over many years. However, this way of looking at PDs carried the implication, widely but mistakenly believed, that these conditions are permanent and incurable. Actually, later research showed that most PD patients improve over time (Skodol et al., 2005; Gunderson et al., 2011), a finding of great clinical importance.

Personality disorder needs to be distinguished, qualitatively and quantitatively, from normal personality. The term "personality" describes traits—that is, patterns of behavior, thought, and emotion that vary between individuals and that are stable and enduring. Psychologists have long been interested in personality, and a whole branch of research (trait psychology) has been developed to study it (John et al., 2008). But the boundary between PD and normal personality is, like most boundaries in psychiatry, fuzzy. This problem sometimes leads clinicians to dismiss the PD construct—along the lines of "Aren't all adolescents a little borderline?" or "Isn't everybody narcissistic?" What such attitudes fail to take into account is that a PD diagnosis is associated with notable effects on functioning (Skodol et al., 2005).

Even so, because PD, like almost everything in DSM, lacks a clear boundary, I consider the prevalence of these conditions (often said to be 10%–15%) to be overestimated (Paris, 2010c). Patients with pervasive and long-term dysfunction in *all* aspects of their lives (both relationships and work) may deserve a diagnosis, but the absence of a clear cut-off supports mission creep. If everyone has a bit of PD, then the diagnosis begins to lose meaning. Even if estimates of 10% prevalence were halved to 5%, we would still be looking at a very common problem.

Personality disorders are an amalgam of traits and symptoms. Although the symptomatic aspects of disorders tend to remit, dysfunctional traits remain stable over time (Skodol et al., 2005; Hopwood et al., 2010). And even when symptoms remit, problematic personality traits persist (Gunderson et al., 2011). For this reason, you cannot make a diagnosis on symptoms alone, as in mood or anxiety disorders. Personality disorders reflect the disruption of higher-order psychological functions, such as motivation, emotional regulation, and behavior. They cannot be reduced to a problem in neurocircuitry or neurochemistry.

For this reason, many researchers on PD have taken a psychological perspective. Until recently, the majority of investigators had a background in psychotherapy rather than psychopharmacology. And to this day, the best evidence for effective treatment in PD supports talking therapy rather than psychopharmacology (Paris, 2008c; Kendall et al., 2009). Yet because PD does not easily fit into the current psychiatric *zeitgeist*, clinicians prefer to go where they believe the "money" is—the symptomatic conditions most likely to respond to drugs. That is why so many clinical reports diagnose major depression and stop there, whereas Axis II is "deferred"—or left blank. As a researcher, I often receive peer review comments on scientific papers asking me to account for comorbidity with depression. In other words, reviewers do not believe that a PD can be independent of mood. Many clinicians have been taught that PD cannot be diagnosed when patients are depressed—in which case one could almost ever make such a diagnosis. However, it has been shown that personality features do not usually remit even when a depression lifts (Lopez-Castroman et al., 2012). Mood disorder is an overvalued but simplistic idea that is often preferred to the more complex construct of PD.

A diagnosis of PD requires longitudinal data. Other conditions in psychiatry, such as substance abuse, also involve chronicity. That has never prevented clinicians from making a diagnosis. And it is not hard to get the kind of information you need. All you have to do is to take a careful history. You can assess life history in an hour, if you know what to ask. But you have to spend the time with patients—something that psychiatrists do less and less these days.

To identify a PD, you need to focus on long-term course rather than on current problems, so a symptom checklist will not do the trick. But if you carefully interview patients, then it is not that difficult to establish whether problems in behavior, emotion, and thinking patterns are stable over time, begin early in life, and have led to dysfunction in multiple contexts. The evaluation needs to establish whether presenting problems are recent or a pattern going back many years. You also need to establish to what extent the problems affect work, relationships, or both. If you cannot obtain sufficient data, interviewing family members can shed light on the life history, making diagnosis more accurate (Zimmerman et al., 1986).

Because patients with personality disorders can be difficult, psychiatrists may dislike them (Lewis & Appleby, 1988). This perception arises from seeing them at their worst, especially in the emergency room, where they so often come with suicidal threats or attempts (Forman et al., 2004). And if patients have prickly and conflictual relationships with other people, the mental health professionals they see will probably not be an exception. Moreover, some patients threaten to commit suicide and imply that if they do so, it will be the therapist's fault. That does not win them much popularity. If patients are truly unpleasant, a negative reaction need not be an example of "countertransference."

Clinicians may have a higher tolerance for psychotic patients, who are, after all, obviously sick—as opposed to nasty. When I tell my colleagues that treating PD is what I do, they offer their condolences. Over the years, many have asked me why I seem to *like* doing most of my clinical work with this population. (Actually, difficult people wake me up in the morning.)

The main reason why clinicians may not diagnose PD is that they think that doing so supports therapeutic pessimism. Recent research has shown this is not true; most patients get better, either with time or with treatment, that the prognosis is actually *better* than in many patients with severe mood and anxiety disorders (Paris, 2008c).

There is also a price to pay for misdiagnosing PDs. Patients with personality disorders are unhappy. That is why they often meet criteria for "comorbid" disorders, such as depression. It is tempting to make mood the focus and to write a quick prescription. That is less than optimal treatment, and overreliance on medication may also do harm.

THE OVERALL DEFINITION OF PERSONALITY DISORDER

DSM-IV introduced a formal definition of personality disorder: an enduring pattern of experience and behavior affecting cognition, affect, interpersonal functioning, and impulse control that is inflexible, pervasive, and leads to clinically significant impairment. (The proposal for DSM-5, now in the Appendix, was more detailed, requiring significant impairments in self and interpersonal functioning, the presence of one or more pathological personality trait domains or trait facets, as well as impairments in personality functioning that are stable across time and consistent across situations.)

Simpler language is needed to convince skeptical clinicians that patients suffer from a PD. (An example is the use of the term "self," which after 40 years in psychiatry, I am still hard put to understand.) On a purely practical level, these patients have lives that don't quite get on track. To pin down that commonsensical concept with reliable observations, clinicians can obtain a history of long-term impairments in relationships and work. Unfortunately, that kind of assessment can be subjective. We should not diagnose every chronically unemployed person with a PD, nor can we always be sure that interpersonal pathology is present, particularly in an era where normal people move from one intimate relationship to another, settle down late, and divorce when unsatisfied. Once again, it is difficult to see where the boundary between normality and impairment lies.

Patients need not be adults to receive PD diagnoses, and DSM-IV allowed for them in adolescents when problems are chronic (except for antisocial PD). Despite hesitancy about diagnosing PDs prior to adulthood, we now know that they begin in adolescence and can be validly diagnosed at that stage (Chanen et al., 2008). One should not downplay serious problems as "adolescent turmoil" that will disappear with maturity.

Should PD be diagnosed in patients whose problems only begin later in life? Not if the definition depends on an early onset followed by a long-term course. People who have functioned reasonably well until their life crashes around them in middle age, and who never recover, probably suffer from a different condition. Although these patients may have problematic personality traits, they managed to get through most of their life.

DIMENSIONALIZATION

Personality disorders were chosen as a "poster child" by the DSM-5 task force leaders to demonstrate the value of scoring as a substitute for categorical psychiatric diagnoses. These proposals were a test case for making DSM-6 and its successors even more dimensional. Moreover, these ideas have long had a large constituency in the personality disorder research community.

A dimensional approach sees personality disorders as dysfunctional amplifications of normal personality profiles. It assumes that there is no fundamental difference between normal and abnormal personality, but a continuum between trait variation and PD that can be seen in both community and clinical populations (Krueger & Bezdjian, 2009). Thus the same measures developed to score normal personality traits could be used to describe disordered personality. It has also been suggested that trait dimensions could allow researchers to determine the "genetic architecture" of PDs through endophenotypes (Livesley, 2011), although the evidence for such a relationship remains slim.

The question is whether dimensionalization is a valid guide to clinical assessment. Moreover, most research has dealt with PDs as categories. Just as light is both a particle and a wave, mental disorders can be both categorical and dimensional. One can artificially square this circle, but only at some cost to reality. In the end, the proposals for DSM-5 were not approved because they downplayed the categories that clinicians find useful and because the dimensional system being proposed had not been thoroughly researched.

Dimensionalization of PD diagnosis may well be reconsidered in DSM-6. But before that can happen, a number of problems will have to be addressed. First, it needs to be recognized that categorical diagnosis can be valid. It is true that PDs, like most categories in nature, have fuzzy boundaries and are not "natural kinds." (Consider, for example, problems with the classification of species in biology.) However, psychopathology is not a smoothly blended continuum but a lumpy pudding. Because of the clumping together of characteristic features, clinicians usually have no trouble distinguishing between normal variations and severe disorders such as psychosis or melancholic depression. Quantitative differences, when striking enough, eventually become qualitative.

Second, most research on PD dimensions is based on observational data, not on etiological or pathogenetic mechanisms. The idea that dimensions correspond to neurobiological reality is a theory that cannot be proven without biological markers.

Third, asking clinicians to score dimensions (mainly by severity) would have been a dicey proposition. Because practitioners are not trained to carry out such ratings, they would very likely be unreliable. It is easier to make self-report scales psychometrically valid, but that takes years.

Fourth, dimensions tell you little about the causes, prevalence, outcome, or treatment of personality disorders. Scores on trait measures do not predict outcome or treatment response. Without that kind of data, one cannot assume that they are more "scientific."

The fifth (and most important) problem with PD dimensions is clinical utility. The procedures proposed for DSM-5 were unfamiliar to most clinicians. This well-intentioned but overly complex dimensional schema would have worked against the recognition of personality disorder. It would have made life for patients suffering from these problems even harder.

Why then have so many researchers in personality disorders advocated dimensionalization? There are several reasons. The first derives from problems with the categorical diagnoses listed in DSM-IV (Livesley, 2011). About half of these categories had little research behind them and were listed mainly because clinicians found them familiar. Second, PD categories overlap with each other. That is mainly because they were described on the basis of clinical tradition, with little effort made to determine the discriminant validity of each criterion. Third, there can be heterogeneity between patients in each category. That is because of a low bar for diagnosis. For example, requiring only five (rather than seven or more) out of nine criteria builds heterogeneity into the system. Finally, about half of the patients who meet overall criteria for a PD could not fit into any category and have to be described as personality disorder, not otherwise specified (Zimmerman et al., 2005). That is a serious problem for any classification, and the one for which dimensional scoring might have been most helpful.

Trait psychologists who wanted PD diagnoses to be made using quantitative scores on trait dimensions have generally favored the Five-Factor Model (FFM; Costa & Widiger, 2001; Widiger, 2011), a system used in thousands of research papers. The FFM describes variations on five broad personality dimensions: (1) extraversion-introversion; (2) neuroticism; (3) openness to experience; (4) agreeableness; and (5) conscientiousness. These factors consistently emerge in studies of community samples and have been shown to be valid across cultures (McCrae & Terracciano, 2005). Other trait schemata measure more or less the same dimensions (Livesley et al., 1998).

But although the FFM does a reasonably good job of describing normal personality, it does not do as well with psychopathology. Ultimately, the data that emerge from factor analysis of questionnaires only reflects what patients say about themselves and needs to be confirmed by behavioral observations as well as biological markers (Huprich et al., 2011). Moreover, dimensional measures can be artificial, given that test construction involves choosing items that measure what theory predicts. Finally, scoring unusually high or low on any trait dimension does not mean a person has a personality disorder (Widiger & Samuel, 2005). People who are highly social (or unsocial), who are highly emotional (or unemotional), who are unusually curious (or uncurious), who are highly agreeable (or disagreeable), or who are highly conscientious (or irresponsible) represent variants of the human condition, not mental disorders. One can only diagnose a PD when traits seriously interfere with functioning and produce significant disability.

Trait scores do give us more information and add color to the black-and-white picture of PD categories. But they tell us more than we need to know for clinical use. They lack the specificity of the classical personality types that every clinician is trained to recognize. Moreover, dimensions lack specificity—for example, almost *all* PD patients are low in agreeableness and conscientiousness (Costa & Widiger, 2001).

Trait profiles are most useful for predicting what type of PD people can develop. Thus highly extraverted people tend to interact in dramatic (histrionic) or demanding (narcissistic) ways, whereas highly introverted (and neurotic) people tend to be afraid of meeting new people (avoidant) or rely on them excessively (dependent). To develop obsessive-compulsive PD, one must already be highly conscientious, whereas people who are unusually low on this trait might develop antisocial PD.

The failure of the PD work group's recommendations for DSM-5 will not heal the split within the PD research community about categories and dimensions. Some support the proposal for a purely dimensional system in ICD-11 (Crawford et al., 2011), which would rate PD by severity and trait profiles alone and eliminate categories entirely. (It remains to see whether this approach will be adopted by ICD, or whether, as happened in DSM-5, it will ultimately be rejected.)

WHY THE PD WORK GROUP'S PROPOSAL WAS REJECTED

The decision of the PD work group to develop its own dimensional model ultimately proved fatal to the enterprise, because it led to a radical revision of diagnostic procedures that was not well backed up by research (as opposed to the FFM). The work group was also seriously split about whether to adopt a purely dimensional model. The members who favored that option were experts in trait psychology, who do not see many patients. Not having seen a large number of cases, these researchers could not relate to the experience of seeing and recognizing characteristic clinical pictures. Work group members who were active clinicians tended to favor categories. The final proposal was a political compromise: a hybrid diagnostic system that used both categories and dimensions to describe personality disorder. But strongly held differences of opinion remained, and two members of the work group resigned in protest.

The outcome was determined both by scientific issues and by politics. The scientific advisory committee to DSM-5, chaired by the eminent psychiatrists Kenneth Kendler and Robert Freeman, concluded that radical changes should not be made without strong evidence. Moreover, the proposals had met political opposition from all sides, particularly from those who were not invited to join the work group. Most trait psychologists favored the well-established FFM and viewed the DSM system as inconsistent with decades of prior research (Widiger, 2011). But most clinicians objected to radical dimensionalization. I signed a letter of protest (along with 31 other experts) defending the use of PD categories in 2011, whereas another group taking the same position published an editorial in the *American Journal of Psychiatry* (Shedler et al., 2010). John Gunderson, the Harvard psychiatrist who had chaired the DSM-IV work group but who was excluded from DSM-5, published his own suggestions for revision (Gunderson, 2010). Other researchers protested the elimination of categories they had been studying for years (e.g., Bornstein, 2011). Zimmerman (2011b, 2012a) noted the absence of a level playing field, given that some retained categories had no research behind them and were as weak scientifically as those that were dropped. Zimmerman (2011b) concluded that the proposed system was almost certain to produce massive unreliability, and Clarkin and Huprich (2011) expressed concern that it would never be used as intended. Allen Frances (2010d), with what turned out to be prescience, recommended retaining the DSM-IV criteria until more evidence was available for change. My own view was that DSM-5 has to have clinical utility and that any system that is overly complex would hurt PD patients by discouraging diagnosis of their condition.

Despite criticism, members of the work group defended their position strongly in scientific journals (Krueger et al., 2011; Skodol et al., 2011). And when I challenged the work group chair (Andrew Skodol) at conferences, his answer was always, "Have you something better?" I didn't. Still, we didn't know enough to change the system. First (2011), as well as Kendler and First (2010), have warned that radical changes in DSM can only be justified by major research breakthroughs. Or as scientists have often said, "Extraordinary claims require extraordinary evidence."

A brief look at the hybrid system proposed for DSM-5 shows how demanding it would have been. It required a series of rating procedures: impairment in personality functioning based on a "Levels of Personality Functioning Scale," a determination whether any of the defined types were present, plus an assessment of 6 trait domains and 29 trait facets. At each step, clinicians would have been asked to use a Likert scale (from 1 to 5) for scoring. Each of these ratings would have required judgment calls to determine what is normal, what is extreme, and what is truly dysfunctional. There was quite a bit of unfamiliar terminology that would be more familiar to researchers than to clinicians. (The idea that DSM should offer different procedures for clinicians and researchers was never seriously considered.) It is safe to conclude that busy clinicians, who have been ignoring the precise instructions of the DSM system for the last three decades, would never have carried out these procedures.

Eliminating Axis II

There is no such thing as "Axis II" in DSM-5 and the five-Axis system as a whole has been eliminated. (There are also no PD "clusters," as described in earlier editions.) DSM-III and DSM-IV had placed the assessment of personality disorders on a separate Axis that was supposed to *encourage* clinicians to pay more attention to PDs. In this respect, Axis II was a complete failure. In fact, the five-Axis system may have made the recognition of PDs *less* likely. Practitioners almost always saw Axis I as the "real" problem and tended to ignore Axis II, which was equated with normal variation. (Insurance companies agreed with this conclusion and did not pay for the treatment of PDs.) In practice, I cannot say how many clinical reports I have read that *only* make an Axis I diagnosis or "deferred" any Axis II diagnosis. As a result of this artificial distinction, PDs remained in an "Axis II ghetto" surrounded by high walls.

DSM-5 rightly decided to classify personality disorders in the same way as every other group in the manual. I doubt that anyone will miss Axis II. The separation of PDs from other mental disorders only made it easier for clinicians to ignore them and to apply other diagnoses that did not lead to specific therapy. If personality disorders are indeed mental disorders—as they surely are—why should they be placed in a different Axis from mood, anxiety, or psychosis? ICD never made this distinction, and most evidence (Roysamb et al., 2011) has supported the conclusion that there is no fundamental difference between symptomatic and personality disorders.

Another good reason for eliminating Axis II is the common perception that personality disorders, unlike symptomatic disorders, are life-long conditions (and incurable). This idea has now been shown to be false—most PDs show remission and recovery over time (Gunderson et al., 2011). In fact, many Axis I disorders are *more* chronic than personality disorders. Finally, Axis II provided an excuse for third parties to refuse payment for the treatment of patients with PDs, no matter how severe. It remains to be seen whether these policies will change in light of DSM-5.

CATEGORIES OF PERSONALITY DISORDER

Another source of controversy in the proposals for DSM-5 was the elimination of 4 of 10 PD categories. This was based on a lack of research on several categories, but some of those retained also had a weak research base.

Like all other diagnoses in the DSM system, PD diagnosis depends on a set of criteria with a cutoff point—the so-called "Chinese menu" approach. But attempts to replace these lists with "prototypes" —that is, several paragraphs describing the common features of each disorder, proved unworkable, as they were lengthy, impossible to remember, and different from the algorithims found everywhere else in the manual. Clinicians wanted PD categories to look like the rest of DSM-5.

1. Antisocial Personality Disorder

Antisocial personality disorder (ASPD) is characterized by manipulativeness, deceitfulness, callousness, and hostility, as well as by disinhibition (irresponsibility, impulsiveness, and risk taking). Robins (1966) and later researchers (Zoccolillo et al., 1992) found that a childhood onset (as conduct disorder) is almost universal. To predict antisociality, the presence of a callous-unemotional specifier for CD is important. Diagnostic inflation could arise from weakening the crucial distinction between childhood vs. adolescent onset of CD, which have very different prognostic implications (Moffitt, 1993).

Psychopathy, a term introduced by Cleckley (1964), is a somewhat different construct, and its large research literature is associated with a standard and widely applied clinical rating scale, the Psychopathy Check List (PCL; Hare, 1993). The ASPD construct has been criticized as being too closely linked to behavior (Hare et al, 1991), as opposed to a more personality-based categorization. Although ASPD is associated with a range of impulsiveness associated with petty criminality, psychopathy is marked by callousness and lack of empathy (Robins, 1966). This construct is of great interest to forensic psychiatry, as it has been used to identify dangerous criminals. Psychopathy is either a different concept from ASPD or a more severe form (Coid & Ullrich, 2010). An attempt in an earlier iteration of DSM-5 to combine the two into one definition was abandoned.

Both antisocial personality and psychopathy have a long history. A hundred years ago the only PD patients recognized as falling within the purview of psychiatry were people sent to hospital after committing crimes. At first, such cases were called "moral insanity," and the patients described by Cleckley (1964) seemed unable to make (or act on) moral judgments.

After ASPD was defined in DSM-III by clear-cut behavioral symptoms, its prevalence was assessed in community populations, and up to 10 years ago, this was the only PD studied by epidemiologists. In the Epidemiological Catchment Area Study (Robins & Regier, 1991), and in later research (Coid et al., 2007) ASPD was found in nearly 3% of the population (mostly males). Antisocial personality disorder is very common in forensic settings. In a recent study (Coid & Ullrich, 2010), it was found in 45% of prisoners, whereas the narrower diagnosis of psychopathy was only identified in 32%.

At this point, the greatest clinical value in diagnosing ASPD may be to identify a group of patients who are *not* treatable. That, of course, could change in the future.

2. Borderline Personality Disorder

The American psychoanalyst Adolf Stern (1938), in a classic paper that is still clinically relevant, was the first writer to use the term "borderline." Until 1980, only antisocial PD had a strong research base, but research on borderline PD (first described in DSM-III) took off, leading to thousands of empirical studies (Paris, 2008b).

The BPD diagnosis is common in practice (Zimmerman et al., 2005), although its precise prevalence depends on the clinical setting. One is most likely to see these patients in the emergency room, with dramatic behaviors that demand attention (e.g., cutting and taking overdoses). They have mood swings that are rapid, are environmentally sensitive, and do not respond well to pharmacological treatment. It is not widely known that about half of BPD patients have quasi-psychotic symptoms, hearing voices under stress, suffering from depersonalization, or showing paranoid thinking. Thus, BPD is a complex disorder that reflects multiple endophenotypes and trait dimensions (Paris, 2007). But complexity leads to overlap and comorbidity, and some researchers (Tyrer et al., 2011; Livesley, 2011) have been suspicious of the diagnosis, preferring to describe these patients as emotionally dysregulated. But that is only part of the clinical picture.

Borderline personality disorder is rooted in affective instability and in impulsive behavioral patterns (Siever & Davis, 1991; Crowell et al., 2009). It is also associated with conflictual and clingy interpersonal relationships (Gunderson, 2007), as well as micropsychotic symptoms. Unfortunately, BPD patients are often given other diagnoses, and personality disorder can be ignored. Many (if not most) are being diagnosed with bipolar disorder. Unfortunately DSM does not address the difference between affective instability and true bipolarity and fails to discriminate BPD from other conditions.

DSM-IV criteria for BPD, never tested for discriminant validity, were insufficiently specific. Research interviews have been developed to make the diagnosis more accurate (Zanarini et al., 1989), describing patients who have *more* than five of nine features listed in earlier manuals. A typical case of BPD, with all features, is unmistakable for any other personality disorder diagnosis.

3. Schizotypal Personality Disorder

It has long been known that patients can have psychotic-like symptoms without crossing the boundary into psychosis. There is a research literature on schizotypal PD (Siever, 2007). In the proposals for DSM-5, the DSM-IV categories of schizoid and paranoid PDs, which reflect less serious symptoms, would have been folded into the schizotypal category. All these patients show negative symptoms of schizophrenia without positive symptoms. The question is whether schizotypy belongs in PDs or in psychoses (where it is cross-listed by DSM-5). These patients have biological markers in common with schizophrenia (Raine et al., 1995), and ICD-10 considers schizotypy a mild form of psychosis. But because this condition rarely progresses to schizophrenia (Siever, 2007), it has been kept in the PD group.

4. Avoidant Personality Disorder

This category was introduced in DSM-III, and ICD-10 developed a similar diagnosis called "anxious personality disorder." However, the category remains poorly studied and has a strong overlap with social phobia (Wakefield et al., 2005). There is very little research on avoidant PD, and some have wondered if it was left in because of its inclusion in the Collaborative Longitudinal Study of Personality Disorders (CLPS; Skodol et al., 2005), a project in which the work group chair was one of the leaders.

5. Obsessive-Compulsive Personality Disorder

Despite its name, this diagnosis should not be confused with OCD. Obsessive-compulsive personality disorder (OCPD) is associated with compulsivity (rigid perfectionism) and negative affectivity (perseveration) but may not present with any symptoms that are recognized by patients. This category has an unclear boundary with normality—one community survey (Grant et al., 2004a) found it in 7% (!) of the population. As clinicians know, compulsive characteristics are generally good in moderation but problematic in excess. Unfortunately, the diagnosis has almost no research behind it. Like avoidant PD, it was included in the CLPS study, which found that like other personality disorders, OCPD improved over time.

6. Narcissistic Personality Disorder

Narcissistic Personality Disorder (NPD) returned from the dead (but by popular demand) in a 2011 revision published on the DSM-5 website, which stated that the work group changed its decision because of feedback indicating that NPD remains a useful clinical construct, as confirmed by a survey (Russ et al., 2008). Most clinicians are familiar with typical cases, and characteristic cases are unmistakable. Although research on NPD is not large, systematic investigation of narcissistic traits has been growing rapidly (Miller et al., 2007; Campbell & Miller, 2011). An article in the New York Times on the subject (Nov 30, 2010) suggested jokingly that narcissists would be upset if the diagnosis had been dropped, because they hate to be ignored—even by DSM. Narcissistic personality disorder is associated with excessive need for approval, grandiosity, entitlement, as well as poor empathy and intimacy. These characteristics make NPD patients uniquely difficult to treat.

OTHER PERSONALITY DISORDER CATEGORIES

In DSM-I and DSM-II, PD diagnoses were a potpourri of ill-defined conditions, and many survived to be included in DSM-III and DSM-IV. Thus the 10 categories in the last edition owed as much to tradition as to science. Four of these old chestnuts were dropped in the DSM-5 proposals. Schizoid personality has not been studied by researchers and may well be a milder form of schizotypal PD (Siever, 2008). Paranoid PD, along with dependent PD, depends on a criteria set describing the same phenomenon eight or nine times in different contexts. (How many ways are there to say "suspicious" or "needy"?) Histrionic PD has no empirical base at all. I am inclined to paraphrase W.S. Gilbert's Lord High Executioner and to conclude, "There's none of them be missed."

Nonetheless, all four have been reinstated along with the DSM-IV system, with the same criteria.

Personality disorder, NOS (or trait specified) can be used for PD patients who do not meet criteria for any category (about half of the total), Because this diagnosis describes a large number of patients, I am rather sorry that formal description by trait profiles has been shelved.

THE GOOD NEWS AND THE BAD NEWS

The inability of DSM-5 to produce a revised system for PDs is an epic story with some overall lessons for the classification of mental disorders. The first is that radical changes require radically new findings. The second is that clinicians are not prepared to give up categories for diagnosis, an approach that dominates all of medicine.

The third problem is that comorbidity is not particular to PDs, but afflicts the DSM system as a whole. Severity makes patients meet criteria for multiple disorders. This is a problem with every category (and group of categories) in the manual. Yet no one has suggested removing major depression because of its enormously high comorbidity with other diagnoses in the manual. In the case of PDs reducing the number of disorders would not have not solved the problem (Zimmerman et al., 2012), which lies in criteria sets that lack discriminant validity. Moreover, there is less comorbidity in community than in clinical samples, as patients have more symptoms (Zimmerman, 2011). The best measure to predict outcome in clinical practice is severity (Hopwood et al, 2011), but severity cannot be rated reliably, as in the staging of tumors or blood pressure.

The fourth issue is that although DSM has too many categories of uncertain validity (Kim & Tyrer, 2010), dimensional ratings are not a solution, because they describe subclinical symptoms that only worsen the problem of diagnostic inflation. As we have seen, that problem afflicts many of the most common and important diagnoses in the manual. Although trait dimensions can add to personality assessment, they are no more "scientific" than categories, as they are also based on self-report or clinical ratings. Nobody has shown that dimensions cut nature at its joints or define the genetic architecture of personality.

Nor has anyone shown that they explain anything about the etiology or pathogenesis of PDs.

Finally, dimensionalization may be less useful for severe PDs than for mild PDs. Trait domains were developed in nonclinical populations, not in patients with severe symptoms. Thus criminality, self-harm, chronic suicidality, and bizarre thoughts are not just exaggerations of normal characteristics but qualitatively different phenomena that most people *never* experience. Traits certainly do not explain why BPD patients have unstable relationships, cut themselves, or overdose when life goes wrong.

Fifth, a diagnostic system *must* have clinical utility. The hybrid system was too complex for practical use, but clinicians never used DSM-IV systematically—not even to make a diagnosis of major depression. Practitioners are busy, often see patients in 10 to 15 minutes, and hardly ever open a manual, whether in book or digital form. To expect them to follow multiple rating procedures virtually guarantees low clinical utility (Rottman et al., 2009; Shedler et al., 2010). Complex procedures only succeed in turning off clinicians, many of whom currently ignore or misdiagnose PDs. The hybrid system was developed by researchers, but it would only have been used by researchers.

THE GAP BETWEEN THEORY AND PRACTICE

The DSM-5 task force insisted that there be no gap between theory and practice in diagnosis. Yet we often know more about treatment of mental disorders than about their etiology. Personality disordered patients can now be managed with success, and that is why it is important to recognize them. Classification will play a crucial role in determining whether these patients receive appropriate and evidence-based treatment or whether they receive multiple pharmacological agents based on poorly conceived diagnoses of mood disorder. Personality disorders need to be on the same level as any other diagnostic group, which is why DSM-III made a mistake in putting them on a separate axis. Using PDs as an experiment in dimensional diagnosis would still have left these conditions in a ghetto.

Few practitioners ever followed the relatively simple algorithims of DSM-III or DSM-IV as directed. I have been teaching the DSM manuals over the last 30 years, but I am the only one I know who counts criteria (which I mainly do to teach residents). Clinicians depend on a gestalt—does this patient look like the picture of some specific diagnosis? In the end, clinicians will shake their heads, and do what they have always done—look for the prototypes already in their minds. This is why categories will continue to dominate diagnosis. They pack a lot of information into a single construct and appeal to busy practitioners who only have a short time to make *any* diagnosis. When I introduced the hybrid system for PDs to psychiatric residents, their reaction was, "Do you really expect us to use this?" No research was conducted to demonstrate the superiority of DSM-5 over DSM-IV.

For psychiatrists like me, who have devoted much of their lives to the study and treatment of PDs, I feel a need for diagnoses that make these conditions easier to identify. In this way I am defending patients. In the end, patients with personality disorders may not be affected by DSM-5. There are too many other reasons for them to be ignored or mistreated.

Chapter 14

Other Diagnostic Groupings

This section will briefly discuss the remaining chapters of DSM-5. All these categories illustrate the same problems that affect the manual as a whole—problems in validating diagnoses and in separating mental disorders from problems in living.

NEUROCOGNITIVE DISORDERS

Psychiatrists see neurocognitive disorders as central to their mandate. In practice, other physicians may identify cases, but the prominent presence of emotional and behavioral symptoms often leaves psychiatrists in charge of treatment. In DSM-IV-TR, these conditions were described as "delerium, dementia, amnestic, and other cognitive disorders." But because dementia, amnestic symptoms, and other signs of brain disease can coexist in the same patients, it makes more sense to apply a common descriptor. (The separate grouping of delerium describes disturbances in awareness and cognition that arise from a medical condition, with specific diagnoses depending on etiology.)

Although cognitive impairment has characteristic clinical features, and a course associated with specific changes in the brain, early diagnosis can be difficult. Sometimes pathology is only definitively identified at autopsy. Often, a differential diagnosis has to be made with mood disorder, which can also lead to loss of concentration and memory. Finally, an early diagnosis does not necessarily change prognosis (Kempler, 1995).

DSM-5 has made a number of changes in classification (Ganguli et al., 2011). This group is now re-labeled as *neurocognitive disorders*. This diagnosis implies a broader and more neutral view about course and disability than "dementia" (which suggests inevitable deterioration). Neurocognitive disorders can take mild or severe forms and are further specified if the etiology is known. Thus, a diagnosis requires decline in one or more cognitive domains (as confirmed by the patient or a reliable informant), confirmation by psychological testing (between 1 and 2 standard deviations below norms for a mild disorder, and 2 or more for a severe disorder), and deficits that interfere with independence.

DSM-5 lists some of the most common causes of neurocognitive disorder, including Alzheimer's, vascular disease, fronto-temporal degeneration, traumatic brain injury, Lewy body disease, Parkinson's, HIV infection, the effects of substance abuse, Huntington's disease, and prion disease. If no cause is known, then a diagnosis of neurocognitive disorder, not elsewhere classified, can be made.

The most important focus of research in recent years has been Alzheimer's disease, which presents with prominent early memory loss and a chronic course. This condition can meet criteria for either mild or severe neurocognitive disorder, depending on the stage of progression. Although "Alzheimer's" remains a subtype, diagnoses in medicine eventually lose their connection to the physician who first described them.

DSM-5 added a category of "mild neurocognitive disorder" to account for cases in which patients have cognitive changes long before anything is visible on a brain scan. But the introduction of the minor type has the potential to create problems. There is no definitive way of distinguishing the effects of aging on memory or attention from an early stage of disorder. Like attenuated psychosis, mild symptoms could be either a precursor of illness or a normal variant. Although a broader definition makes false–negatives less likely, it makes false–positives more likely. The danger is that people with normal cognitive changes will be given an incorrect (and alarming) diagnosis. DSM-5 runs the danger of classifying aging itself as pathological.

The problem would be resolved if we had biological markers that could be measured early in the course of illness. But neuroimaging findings appear too late, and we need a marker that can be identified earlier and that reliably predicts a deteriorating course. That remains a task for the future. It also remains to be seen whether the revised system in DSM-5 will have greater clinical utility than its predecessors.

Rabins and Lyketsos (2011), reviewing the changes in DSM-5, were generally supportive. If there is no absolute requirement for memory impairment, then the diagnosis can be made through a wide range of effects. DSM-5 also requires the use of a standardized procedure, which could be either a mini-mental status or a psychological test to confirm a deficit. It is always better to have a measure that is at least partly independent of clinical observation. I only wish that this principle had been applied more generally in the DSM manual.

In summary, the new system is not difficult to use. The problem is that like many other revisions in the manual, it introduces a severity-based and dimensional approach to diagnosis that tends to identify false–positives.

SOMATIC SYMPTOM DISORDER

Somatic symptoms are poorly understood orphans in the diagnostic classification. Chronic fatigue and pain are among the most common complaints of patients described in the past as "psychosomatic" (Shorter, 1993, 1994). Although research on unexplained physical symptoms in medicine has been thin, when patients present in this way, physicians in primary care often send them to psychiatrists for evaluation and treatment. (It is usually not the patient who initiates the referral but the doctor, after a series of unfruitful investigations.)

In the past, somatic syndromes were described as "hysteria"—a perjorative and misleading term that dates back to Hippocrates. Later, symptoms that resembled neurological conditions were called "conversion," a Freudian term that was retained in DSM-IV, now changed to *functional neurological symptom disorder*. The criteria for this new diagnosis no longer include, as did previous editions, the difficult-to-prove statement that psychological conflict lies behind these symptoms. Other patients present with medically unexplained pain, a syndrome considered a diagnosis in its own right by DSM-IV (but not by DSM-5). Other patients constantly worry about being sick, which earned them a DSM-IV diagnosis of *hypochondriasis* (another term associated with Hippocrates). Most of these patients can now be diagnosed with *illness anxiety disorder.*

The new category of *somatic symptom disorder* (SSD) includes many patients previously diagnosed with somatization disorder, hypochondriasis, and pain disorder and can be coded for severity. Another category, important for consultation-liaison psychiatry, is *psychological factors affecting medical conditions.* The rare entity of *factitious disorder* describes patients who fake physical disorders. Psychiatrists may see these cases in consultation, and they are included under SSDs (Krahn et al., 2008), although these patients are *consciously* pretending to be sick. It also has the twist that some cases involve other people, such as children, leading to the concept of "Munchausen's by proxy." Finally, body dysmorphic disorder, which was in this group in DSM-IV, has been moved to the OCD spectrum.

The DSM-5 approach offers a simplification of a complex system that clinicians found hard to use. Somatization disorder, a term introduced in DSM-III, described a picture marked by multiple physical complaints over many years and was studied and described by psychiatrists at Washington University in St. Louis but was uncommon in other settings. Epidemiological research using DSM-IV definitions has confirmed that this entity is rare, with prevalence estimated at 0.2% (Kessler et al., 2005). Among the many thousands of consults I have conducted over the last 40 years, I can remember seeing only a few cases. Moreover, the construct of somatization disorder was idiosyncratic, restrictive, and tended to reinforce a mind–body dichotomy.

In summary, SSDs can be divided into *complex somatic symptom disorder* (CSSD; multiple symptoms, excessive concern about health, chronicity), *simple somatic symptom disorder* (one main symptom with duration of at least one month), *illness anxiety disorder,* and *functional neurological disorder.* Subcategories describe cases in which somatic complaints, hypochondriasis, and pain are most prominent.

Rief et al. (2011) found that DSM-5 diagnoses of somatic syndromes remained stable over a 1-year period. But the specific symptoms that patients present vary with time and place. They are a function of a social "symptom pool" and reflect ways in which social forces shape the way patients experience distress (Shorter, 1993). Most people express distress through the body, and in many cultures, dysphoric emotions such as depression present as fatigue or pain rather than as mental states (Kleinman, 1991).

DISSOCIATIVE DISORDERS

Although somatic symptom disorders are common, dissociative disorders are uncommon—so uncommon, in fact, that they may not even exist (Lynn et al., 2012).

More than a hundred years ago, the French psychiatrist Pierre Janet coined the term *dissociation* to describe a state of mind in which different aspects of identity become separated, splitting consciousness to make some parts of memory and personality unavailable to other parts (Carroy & Plas, 2000). Dissociation is a dramatic phenomenon that has fascinated the general public—as well as some mental health professionals. Psychologist Morton Prince (1906) wrote a book describing a patient with multiple personalities. Fifty years later, "The Three Faces of Eve" (Thigpen & Cleckly, 1957) became a best-seller that was turned into a successful Hollywood movie. In the 1970s, the theory that dissociation into multiple personalities results from child abuse was popularized in another best-seller, "Sibyl" (Schreiber, 1973). This book was at least partly responsible for an epidemic of diagnosis of multiple personality disorder (Piper & Merskey, 2004).

Rieber (2006) has shown that the case history of Sibyl (real name Shirley Mason) was a fabrication. The story was created by a troubled but compliant patient, an over-enthusiastic therapist, and an author looking to make money. Sibyl invented her multiple personalities—as well a history of child abuse that claimed to explain them—to please her therapist, Cornelia Wilbur, who found a journalist (Flora Schreiber) to write the book. These conclusions have been confirmed by examining all documents in the case, showing that Shirley Mason's childhood was normal (Nathan, 2011).

Multiple personality (now relabeled as "dissociative identity disorder," or DID) is an artifact brought on by suggestive therapy techniques

(Piper & Merskey, 2004). Patients are actively encouraged to present additional personalities, and hypnosis is used to elicit them. These procedures do not produce dissociative phenomena in everyone but can do so in susceptible patients. Dissociation is a common symptom in other mental disorders but can be reinforced when therapists become fascinated with it.

The claim that dissociation results from childhood trauma is doubtful. Most people who were abused as children never develop such symptoms, and therapies that aim to uncover putatively repressed traumatic events make use of hypnosis, a technique that elicits dramatic stories and false memories (Paris, 1996). The concept of repressed memories of trauma has led to a rash of accusations against families, and for a while, working in a daycare center sometimes threatened to become a high-risk occupation.

Up to a few decades ago, these conditions were considered very rare. They were included in the classification system only after being described in medical journals. In DSM-II, dissociative disorders were as a subtype of "hysterical neurosis." But, with the demise of both terms ("hysteria" *and* "neurosis") in DSM-III, dissociative disorders were orphaned. The paradoxical result was that they had to be placed in a separate grouping. That decision proved fateful. Ever since 1980, as textbooks of psychiatry felt required to follow the DSM system, each version has had a chapter on dissociative disorders.

Most psychiatrists never make diagnoses of dissociative disorders, and most have never seen a case. But a group of mavens and true believers promoted the concept. Textbook chapters are written by these "experts," whereas psychiatrists who believed the diagnoses were a serious mistake unsuccessfully lobbied for their elimination.

Sometimes it takes only one powerful voice to determine what gets in, or stays in, the DSM manual. In this case, the voice belongs to the influential Stanford psychiatrist David Spiegel, who has promoted dissociative disorders for decades (Spiegel, 1994). There was no chance of a change once a task force was struck that included Spiegel. Those who recommended elimination of the group were ignored. The DSM-5 approach to dissociative disorders (Spiegel et al., 2011) offers only minor revisions.

We all have to live with DSM-5, so textbooks will continue to have a chapter on dissociative disorders, and psychiatric residency programs will have to teach trainees about it. Few are willing to say that these conditions are, at best, rare and, at worst, mythical. One can only hope that once the proponents of DID have passed from the scene, the diagnosis will wither away with time.

Although the syndrome of multiple personality is an artifact of therapeutic suggestion, trance and possession states are not. They are common ways of expressing distress in some cultural groups (During et al., 2011). These conditions, even if they are syndromes, could find a place in another chapter of the manual.

Contrary to the drama that has driven the epidemic of multiple personality disorder, there is no consistent relationship between trauma and dissociation (Lynn et al., 2012). Rather a capacity to dissociate in specific patients can be exaggerated by social forces, which is what happened in the 1990s.

SLEEP–WAKE DISORDERS

This group of disorders was absent from DSM-III and only introduced to the manual in DSM-IV. How did practitioners manage without them until 1994? Most anomalies of sleep seen in psychiatric practice are associated with other diagnoses (Breslau et al., 1996). However, some sleep disorders are not associated with other mental disorders. These syndromes are uncommon and belong less to psychiatry than to neurology. The detailed criteria in DSM-IV were therefore written for subspecialists who run sleep clinics. Speaking on behalf of the work group, Reynolds and Redline (2010) have suggested that the new classification in DSM-5 will be user-friendly for general psychiatrists. It is hard to see how this could be true.

The categories of sleep–wake disorders include primary insomnia, hypersomnolence, narcolepsy/hypocretin disorders, obstructive sleep apnea hypopena disorder, central sleep apnea, sleep-related hypoventilation, set of circadian rhythm sleep disorders, disorder or arousal, nightmare disorder, rapid eye movement sleep behavior disorder, restless leg syndrome, and substance-induced sleep disorder. These are all rare syndromes, and a few are new categories. This shows how the DSM process works. Specialists tend to be splitters rather than lumpers. Because most psychiatrists pay less attention to this chapter, diagnoses can proliferate without objection.

ELIMINATION DISORDERS

As anyone knows who tries to maintain a filing system, all classification systems break down at some point, leaving a large number in a "miscellaneous" group. DSM has a separate chapter that includes two diagnoses seen in children: enuresis and encopresis. These problems are not even syndromes but symptoms. They were included because some cases have no obvious cause. The manual presents one caveat—enuresis should only be diagnosed when it does not result from a medical condition.

SUICIDAL BEHAVIOR DISORDER

Even after listing "left-over" symptoms, DSM-5 still has its own chapter of "other" disorders. Non-suicidal self-injury (NSSI) is a behavioral pattern introduced because it represents a common symptom not explained by other diagnoses. There has been a recent increase in the prevalence of NSSI among adolescents (Lloyd-Richardson et al., 2007). Cutting oneself on the wrist (or less visible areas) is not usually suicidal behavior but functions as a means of regulating negative affects (Linehan, 1993). Some adolescents who self-harm develop borderline personality disorder, associated with unstable mood, unstable relationships, and other forms of impulsivity (Chanrn et al., 2008). Most simply experiment with cutting, driven by social contagion (Winchel & Stanley, 1991), and most remit when followed over time (Moran et al., 2012).

To avoid drawing firm conclusions about the meaning of these behaviors, DSM-5 had proposed a category whose criteria required self-injury on 5 days or more in the past year without suicidal intent and associated with an attempt to deal with negative affect. When this concept proved unreliable in field trials it was replaced in 2012 by *suicidal behavioral disorder*. Yet the necessity for such a category was not clear. Defining a mental disorder by a few symptoms, no matter how common, goes against all the principles of nosology. The diagnosis was eventually left in the Appendix for further study.

ADJUSTMENT DISORDERS

This group was introduced in DSM-III to describe conditions in which patients experienced symptomatic reactions to stressors but did not meet criteria for any mental disorder. The reaction to a stressor needs to be somewhat exaggerated but is defined as temporary, going away when the stressor goes away (or at least within 6 months after exposure).

It is difficult to determine what is a normal reaction to a stressful event and a disorder. But adjusting to stress is not an illness. I also find that some clinicians invoke this category whenever something difficult is going on in a patient's life, even if they meet criteria for a more substantive diagnosis. (In DSM-IV, stressors were coded on Axis IV.)

Adjustment disorders are normal variants. The category may have been kept in the manual to justify seeing these patients in consultation or treatment. But this kind of categorization runs the risk of medicalizing life itself.

PATIENTS WITH NO MENTAL DISORDER

Believe it or not, there are still patients who come to clinical attention without meeting criteria for *any* disorder listed in DSM. Nonetheless, a diagnostic code may have to be provided when insurance requires one.

The "V codes" listed at the end of the manual are designed to describe consultations for life problems that are *not* disorders. The list includes marital strife, conflict with children, and unemployment. Obviously, all these problems can occur in people who do have mental disorders.

Proposals to add a new group to the manual, called "relational disorders" (Beach et al., 2006), were motivated more by insurance than by science. Psychiatrists who practice marital and family therapy wanted to have their work validated by a diagnosis. Others, who practice psychotherapy to treat life problems were in the same position. If this idea had been accepted, then it might have achieved the goal of making the prevalence of mental disorder in the population 100%. However, this group did not find its way into DSM-5.

A WORD IN SUMMARY

This brings us to the end of our survey of DSM-5 diagnoses. Obviously, the classification of mental disorders is far from hard science. It is a rough-and-ready way of making sense of a wide variety of conditions. This is a necessary task, but we need not see DSM categories as "real." Some diagnoses in the manual would be recognized as illnesses by almost anyone. Others continue to be controversial, largely because they medicalize the human condition. We need to keep in mind that DSM is not a "bible" but a work in progress.

PART III

OVERVIEW

Chapter 15

A Guide for the Perplexed

I have borrowed the title of this chapter from a famous book by the twelfth century religious philosopher Moses Maimonides. Although the DSM manual is not concerned with morality or religion, it has sometimes been treated as a sacred text. The media like to refer to it as "psychiatry's bible." Yet what the DSM manuals represent is only the opinion of a group of experts, published by one professional organization at one specific time in history. When one examines how mental disorders were defined in the past, many categories and concepts are outdated. That is how current manuals will look in a few decades. We should be humble and accept our ignorance.

If you were to believe the hype, DSM-5 has taken a dramatic step into the future. Actually, diagnosis is not radically different from DSM-IV—it just continues a long-term trend of expansion into the realm of normality. But DSM-5 does not offer a paradigm shift. That was the only possible option—psychiatry should not and cannot make radical revisions until it learns more about the etiology of mental illness (Kendler & First, 2010; First, 2010). Any claim that DSM-5 is based on better science than its predecessors is dubious.

Research is nowhere near to solving the problems at the core of mental illness. Most psychiatric diagnoses remain syndromes. Thirty-odd years after DSM-III, we are still in the dark about the nature of most disorders that psychiatrists treat. We have a lot more data, but their interpretation remains controversial. Advances in neuroscience have not succeeded in explaining any mental disorder. Genetics has raised more questions than it can answer. Neurochemistry turns out to be much more complex than most people believed. And the beautiful pictures of neuroimaging will be seen by future generations as, at best, suggestive and, at worst, primitive. Clinical observation and consensus from experts, rather than hard facts, are still the guiding forces behind the manual. Without more basic knowledge, there was really no alternative.

THE IMPACT OF DSM-5 ON MENTAL HEALTH CARE

Psychiatry has changed in the last few decades, and the various editions of DSM have been part of that change. The field has moved very far from its previous identification with talking therapy, and biological psychiatry dominates theory and practice. However, this has not been a boon for patients, many of whom now receive a 15-minute check-up in which medications are reviewed and "adjusted." This kind of practice does not allow psychiatrists enough time to find out what is going on in a patient's life (Carlat, 2010).

DSM-5's ideology supports all these trends. The practice that follows from a reductionistic view of psychiatry presents itself as a clinical application of neuroscience. In other words, drugs and more drugs. This need not necessarily follow, because a neuroscience perspective remains compatible with a broader range of interventions. But practitioners like diagnoses that lead directly to pharmacological interventions. Typically, patients diagnosed with psychosis get an antipsychotic, those diagnosed with bipolar disorder get a mood stabilizer, those diagnosed with depression get an antidepressant, and those diagnosed with attention-deficit hyperactivity disorder (ADHD) get a stimulant. Some patients can be prescribed all of these agents. On the surface, these procedures resemble those of internal medicine. A closer look shows that they are not evidence-based (Paris, 2010a).

The most important issue for DSM-5 is the expansion of diagnostic boundaries. Although the most typical cases of any disorder often respond to specific treatment interventions, patients who only have *some* symptoms corresponding to a diagnostic category may not. For example, although patients with classical features of schizophrenia almost always respond to antipsychotics, patients with attenuated symptoms may not. Although patients with melancholic depression often respond to antidepressants, patients with mild depressive symptoms may not. Although patients with classical bipolar-I disorder usually do well with lithium, patients with "bipolar spectrum disorders" may not. Although patients with classical ADHD often improve on stimulants, those who have attention problems resulting from other causes may not.

DSM-5, by expanding the definition of most disorders in the manual, encourages over-treatment. It is bad enough that standards of care have deteriorated to the point that drugs are often used off-label, with antipsychotics routinely used to treat anxiety (Comer et al., 2011). But broadened diagnostic criteria will be used to justify prescribing drugs to patients who are unlikely to benefit from them.

We are told, without solid evidence, that millions of people with mental symptoms are tragically undertreated. Again, the subtext is drugs. Although it is true that some patients with severe disorders are not getting the help they need, mild or subclinical symptoms may not need the same treatment or any treatment at all. The thrust of these arguments, usually based on epidemiological data, is that drugs should be prescribed to an even larger percentage of the population than is already the case. The pharmaceutical industry can only rejoice at such conclusions. The rest of us are left to weep.

I am impressed with how much patients have bought into this story. They are the ultimate consumers of DSM-5 and have been convinced that the diagnoses offered to them are *real*. They do not know that some are, but that most are not. I have carried out thousands of consultations for patients seen in primary care, most of whom will have already received a DSM diagnosis. Patients become attached to these labels, telling me with conviction, "I have been *diagnosed* with (depression, bipolar disorder, ADHD)." They use the word as if it were based on scientific procedures, much like a medical diagnosis. Some even ask me if they can have a blood test or a brain scan to confirm what they have already been told. Some have faith in psychological testing (now the most common way to "confirm" a diagnosis of ADHD) or in rating scales (sometimes used to place patients in a bipolar spectrum).

In this way, the DSM system has become part of patient culture. I cannot fault people for wanting to believe that psychiatric diagnosis is precise and scientific and that it leads to specific and evidence-based treatment. But they are wrong, even if DSM-5 encourages them to think so.

DSM-5 AND SOCIETY

Mental health practitioners are not the only people who read diagnostic manuals. Patients, lawyers, and the educated public can be expected to take a close look at DSM-5. Although I am concerned that patients will see the manual as scientifically proven, there is a benefit to having the criteria for diagnoses readily available on the Internet. I tell my patients to read up on their condition, so they can discuss diagnosis and treatment planning more intelligently.

The use of DSM-5 by the courts worries me more. Although it has long been accepted that criminal responsibility is not possible in people with psychotic delusions, the law's adversarial system will always tempt some lawyers to present a defense on psychiatric grounds, particularly when there is no doubt that a crime has been committed. I often see patients with personality disorders who have been arrested for shoplifting but do not want to face the consequences of a conviction. In some cases, a diagnosis of depression has even been used as a successful defense in murder cases.

The civil law is even more likely to be affected. In custody disputes, the courts consider all kinds of diagnoses and accept all kinds of psychiatric testimony. The perception that DSM-5 diagnoses are "real," and that experts know how to make them, has created these problems. Yet there is no empirical evidence that diagnoses explain much about the kinds of human behavior that end up involving the legal system.

Finally, I am concerned about how the educated public will receive DSM-5. Over-expansion of diagnosis is sometimes ridiculed in the media, feeding into anti-psychiatric critiques of real diagnoses, such as psychoses. I can only hope that the public will understand that diagnostic manuals are pragmatic systems and do not correspond to Platonic truth. The experience of the last 30 years shows that once diagnoses are in the manual, they become reified and treated with reverence. I would like to see the media, and the public they serve, be more critical of DSM-5 than they were of past editions.

HOW CLINICIANS SHOULD USE DSM-5

Fortunately, clinicians are pragmatic. They did not take any of the previous manuals as gospel and will not do so this time. They use diagnosis in ways perceived to have implications for treatment. My advice is to work with the current criteria as much as possible but to decline to apply them rigidly where they do not make sense.

For decades, we have treated DSM as if it contained scientific truth, rather than what it really is—a rough draft based on expert consensus. The manual remains the main guide to psychiatry for medical students and residents. But its mechanical approach to diagnosis and treatment is not appropriate for sophisticated medical specialists. Psychiatry has a richer diagnostic tradition that should trump constructs that are little but political compromises. I have taught the DSM system to students and residents for more than 40 years. My advice has consistently been— *learn it but don't believe in it.* My recommendation to clinicians using DSM-5 is precisely the same.

PREPARING FOR DSM-6

Judging by the history of past editions, DSM-5 should, like DSM-IV, last for at least 15 years. It is possible that regular revisions will be released, as suggested by the use of Arabic rather than Roman numerals, but given the controversy and disruption that accompanies even the most minor changes, I am skeptical. Unless important scientific discoveries emerge in the coming years, DSM-5.1 or DSM-5.2 can only make only minor revisions. If DSM-6 is published in 2028, I am unlikely to live to see it. But there are several issues we already know the next edition will have to address.

The first, emphasized throughout this book, is the relationship between mental disorder and normality. Up to now, each edition has expanded the range of psychiatric diagnosis. That process cannot continue indefinitely. When textbooks get too large, people stop using them. At some point one has to set a limit. The vision of DSM-5 fails to acknowledge this boundary. Mental disorder is seen as a point on a continuum between no symptoms (rarely), subclinical symptoms (very commonly), and clinically significant symptoms (less common). This point of view medicalizes the human condition.

Thus the greatest flaw in DSM-5 is an expansive pathologizing of life experiences. One can't help thinking again of the quip that: "Life is the disease and psychiatry is the cure." Our specialty would gain more respect if it confined itself to conditions that everyone agrees are mental disorders. Rather, the boundaries between disorder and normality have been widened to include "subclinical" problems that could just as easily be viewed as part of the human condition. This tendency can be seen in expansions of the psychoses, of bipolarity, the downgrading of exclusions for depression, and over-inclusive concepts of ADHD, autism, and addiction.

Although biology tends to blur the difference between the subclinical and the clinical, as in the distinction between a narrowed coronary artery and a myocardial infarct, we live most of our lives in variable states of health, without necessarily feeling we suffer from disease. The neo-Kraepelinian model may not be a perfect model of psychopathology, but it is based on the idea that mental illness is unusual rather than ubiquitous.

To address the issue, I hope that biological markers will eventually be found to make more valid diagnoses. Markers could also be used to define a clinically meaningful cut-off point (as in hypertension). In addition, they could be used to determine whether symptoms that look similar actually fall within the same spectrum. Yet in all of these cases, expansion of diagnosis should be tamed until we can identify biological correlates and quantify them.

Some think that by the time DSM-6 is published, biological measures will be sufficiently specific that they will be used directly as diagnostic criteria. (Once again, we keep hearing about breakthroughs just around the corner.) But I doubt this will happen by 2028. And even where markers turn out to be helpful, they measure risk factors rather than illness itself. That is why psychiatry needs to retain a biopsychosocial approach to mental disorders. Although further progress in diagnosis will involve closer links with neurobiology, psychiatry needs to continue studying mental experiences and psychological symptoms in their own right. It will never be possible to completely reduce mental phenomena to a cellular or chemical level.

This raises another challenge for DSM-6—developing better psychometrics for the assessment of psychopathology. This cannot be done in the "quick and dirty" way that DSM-5 suggests, asking busy clinicians to carry out ratings that may or may not be reliable. Measuring symptoms systematically requires years of research.

The expansiveness of DSM-5 also carries risks for the mental health system. It already has its hands full managing a large number of severely ill patients whose illness no one would deny. It does not need to take on the care of additional millions of people who have subclinical symptoms and who may not require specialized services at all. Moreover, third parties may not pay for treatment if everyone is made eligible.

DSM-5 remains a book of considerable size. Because the manual is available on the Web, one no longer needs to carry around a heavy book. Even so, DSM-5 is long. Expansion has been continuous since 1952 and has not stopped. As Horwitz, (2002, p. 80) sagely noted: "Once a diagnosis has been created, it enters professional curricula, specialists emerge to treat it, conferences are organized around it, research and publications deal with it, careers are built around it, and patients formulate their symptoms to correspond to it."

The antidote to these poisons is to apply extra caution and follow common sense. The manual leaves us some latitude, because DSM-5 continues to require that all diagnostic criteria attain "clinical significance." Unfortunately it also leaves latitude to do the opposite and turn the human condition into a set of diagnoses.

A second and related problem concerns situations in which lowering a diagnostic threshold leads directly to the introduction of therapy whose evidence base has not been established in a wider population.

For me the most troubling example is the diagnosis of "bipolar spectrum disorder," leading to prescription of mood stabilizers and/or antipsychotic drugs. Exercising caution in such cases could save many patients from unnecessary pharmacological regimes with all their attendant side effects.

DSM-5 is a provisional manual that allows clinicians to communicate with each other. That is why revising it only every 15 years is wise. But a more basic understanding of mental illness lies many decades away. DSM-6 will come too soon to provide answers.

FINAL THOUGHTS

I have to ask myself, after writing a book-length critique, whether the revision of the DSM manual could have been done differently. The answer is yes. First, although recognizing the need for revision, it should have been carried out with more humility and been incremental rather than reach for a paradigm change that cannot justified by the current state of evidence. Second, although psychiatry cannot do without a diagnostic system describing categories of disorder, we do not need so many of them, with each edition adding on more. If the main purpose of the manual is to guide clinical work, then it could have been made much simpler. Third, DSM-5 has been misled by its faith in neuroscience to expand diagnosis unjustifiably, diagnosing life itself. Doing so can only bring the manual into disrepute.

I support the DSM system as a broad concept. It is better to have a flawed classification than none at all. I remember the chaos of DSM-I and DSM-II, which were theoretically unsound and provided little or no clinical guidance. DSM-5 is a noble attempt, but without a knowledge of underlying disease processes, its classification of mental disorder can only be provisional.

To practice, to teach, or to do research, mental health professionals need to be humble. They should see themselves as part of a great chain stretching from past to future. Science (and the application of science) is a journey, but those who embark never quite arrive. This is how we should view DSM-5. It attempts to do the best it can without the knowledge required to reach solid conclusions about the nature of mental illness. We have to look to the future for the kind of understanding that would allow us to develop an evidence-based classification. Until then, DSM-5 could remain much like Winston Churchill's comment on democracy: the worst possible diagnostic system—except for any other yet devised.

REFERENCES

Abrams, R, Taylor, MA. (1981): Importance of schizophrenic symptoms in the diagnosis of mania. *American Journal of Psychiatry* 138:658–661.

Addington, J, Epstein, I, Reynolds, A, Furimsky, I, Rudy, L, Mancini, B, et al. (2008): Early detection of psychosis: finding those at clinical high risk, *Early Intervention in Psychiatry* 2:147–153.

Agrawal, A, Heath, AC, Lynskey, MT. (2011): DSM-IV to DSM-5: the impact of proposed revisions on diagnosis of alcohol use disorders. *Addiction.* 106:1935–1943.

Akiskal, HS. (2002): The bipolar spectrum: the shaping of a new paradigm in psychiatry. *Current Psychiatry Reports* 4: 1–3.

Akiskal, HS, Akiskal, KK, Lancrenon, S, Hantouche, EG, Fraud, J-P, Gury, C, et al. (2006): Validating the bipolar spectrum in the French National EPIDEP Study: overview of the phenomenology and relative prevalence of its clinical prototypes. *Journal of Affective Disorders* 96:197–205.

Akiskal, HS, McKinney, WT Jr. (1973): Depressive disorders: toward a unified hypothesis. *Science* 182:20–29.

American Psychiatric Association. (1952): *Diagnostic and Statistical Manual of Mental Disorders.* Washington, DC: Author.

American Psychiatric Association. (1968): *Diagnostic and Statistical Manual of Mental Disorders* (2nd ed.).Washington, DC: Author.

American Psychiatric Association. (1980): *Diagnostic and Statistical Manual of Mental Disorders* (3rd ed.).Washington, DC: Author.

American Psychiatric Association. (1987): *Diagnostic and Statistical Manual of Mental Disorders*, revised (3rd ed.). Washington, DC: Author.

American Psychiatric Association. (1994): *Diagnostic and Statistical Manual of Mental Disorders* (4th ed.). Washington, DC: Author.

American Psychiatric Association. (2000): *Diagnostic and Statistical Manual of Mental Disorders*, text revision (4th ed.). Washington, DC: Author.

Andrews, G, Charney, DS, Sirovatka, PJ, Regier, DA (eds). (2009): *Stress-Induced and Fear Circuitry Disorders: Refining the Research Agenda for DSM-5*. Arlington VA: American Psychiatric Association.

Amminger, GP, Schäfer MR, Papageorgiou K, Klier, CM, Cotton SM, Harrigan, SM, et al. (2010): Long-chain omega-3 fatty acids for indicated prevention of psychotic disorders: a randomized, placebo-controlled trial. *Archives of General Psychiatry*. 67:146–154.

Anatchkova, MD, Bjorner, JB. (2010): Health and role functioning: the use of focus groups in the development of an item bank. *Quality of Life Research* 19:111–123.

Andreasen, NC. (1979): Affective flattening and the criteria for schizophrenia. *American Journal of Psychiatry*. 136:944–947.

Andrews, G, Hobbs, MJ. (2010): The effect of the draft DSM-5 criteria for GAD on prevalence and severity. *Australian and New Zealand Journal of Psychiatry*. 44:784–790.

Angell, M. (2000): Is academic medicine for sale? *NEJM*. 342:1516–1518.

Angst, J. (1998): The emerging epidemiology of hypomania and bipolar II disorder. *Journal of Affective Disorders*. 50:143–151.

Angst, J, Gamma, A. (2002): A new bipolar spectrum concept: a brief review. *Bipolar Disorders* 4:11–14.

Angst, J, Merikangas, K. (1997): The depressive spectrum: diagnostic classification and course. *Journal of Affective Disorders*. 45:31–39.

Balint, GP, Buchanan, WW, Dequeker, J. (2006): A brief history of medical taxonomy and diagnosis. *Journal of Clinical Rheumatology*. 25:132–135.

Batstra, L, Frances, AJ. (2012): DSM-5 further inflates Attention Deficit Hyperactivity Disorder. *Journal of Nervous and Mental Diseases*. 200:486–488.

Beach, SR, Wamboldt, MZ, Kaslow, NJ, Heyman, RE, First, MB. Underwood, LG, et al. (2006): *Relational Processes and DSM-V: Neuroscience, Assessment, Prevention, and Treatment*. Arlington, Virginia: American Psychiatric Publishing.

Beautrais, AL. (2001): Suicides and serious suicide attempts: two populations or one? *Psychological Medicine*. 31:837–845.

Beck, AT, Resnik, L, Lettieri, DJ. (1974): *The Prediction of Suicide*. Bowie, MD: Charles Press.

Beck, AT, Steer, RA, Brown, GK. (1996): *BDI-II manual*. San Antonio, TX: The Psychological Corporation, Harcourt Brace and Co.

Benazzi, F. (2002): Highly recurrent unipolar may be related to bipolar II. *Comprehensive Psychiatry.* 43:263–268.

Benazzi, F. (2004): Factor structure of recalled DSM-IV hypomanic symptoms of bipolar II disorder. *Comprehensive Psychiatry* 45:441–446.

Benes, FM. (2010): Searching for unique endophenotypes for schizophrenia and bipolar disorder within neural circuits and their molecular regulatory mechanisms. In Tamminga, C, Sirovatka, PJ, Regier, DA, van Os, J. (Eds.). *Deconstructing Psychosis: Refining the Research Agenda for DSM-V.* Washington DC: American Psychiatric Press, pp. 99–108.

Bentall, RP, Rowse, G, Shryane, N, Kinderman, P. (2009): The cognitive and affective structure of paranoid delusions: a transdiagnostic investigation of patients with schizophrenia spectrum disorders and depression. *Archives of General Psychiatry.* 66:236–247.

Berganza, CE, Mezzich, JE, Pouncey, C. (2005): Concepts of disease: Their relevance for psychiatric diagnosis and classification. *Psychopathology;* 38:166–170.

Berrios, GE. (1993): European views on personality disorders: A conceptual history. *Comprehensive Psychiatry* 34:14–30.

Bienvenu, OJ, Samuels, JF, Wuyek, A, Liang, K-Y, Wang, Y, Grados, MA, et al. (2011): Is obsessive-compulsive disorder an anxiety disorder and what, if any, are spectrum conditions: a family study perspective. *Psychological Medicine* DOI:10.1017/S0033291711000742

Birmaher, B, Axelson, D. (2006): Course and outcome of bipolar spectrum disorder in children and adolescents: a review of the existing literature. *Development & Psychopathology* 18:1023–1035.

Birmaher, B, Axelson, D, Goldstein, B, Brent, D, Kupfer, D. (2010): Psychiatric Disorders in Preschool Offspring of Parents With Bipolar Disorder: The Pittsburgh Bipolar Offspring Study (BIOS). *American Journal of Psychiatry;* 167:321–330.

Birmaher, B, Axelson, D, Goldstein, B, Strober, M. (2009): Four-year longitudinal course of children and adolescents with bipolar spectrum disorders: The Course and Outcome of Bipolar Youth (COBY) Study. *American Journal of Psychiatry* 166:795–804.

Blanchard, R. (2005): Early history of the concept of autogynephilia. *Archives of Sexual Behavior* 34:439–446.

Blashfield, R, Livesley, WJ. (1999): Classification. In Millon, T, Blaney, PH, Davis, RD (Eds.). *Oxford Textbook of Psychopathology.* New York: Oxford University Press, pp. 3–28.

Block, JJ. (2008): Issues for DSM-V: Internet Addiction. *American Journal of Psychiatry* 165:306–307.

Bongar, B. (1992): *Suicide: Guidelines for Assessment, Management, and Treatment.* New York: Oxford University Press.

Bornstein, R. (2011): Reconceptualizing personality pathology in DSM-5: Limitations in Evidence for Eliminating Dependent Personality Disorder and Other DSM-IV syndromes. *Journal of Personality Disorders* 25:235–247.

Breslau, N, Davis, GC, Andreski, P. (1991): Traumatic events and posttraumatic stress disorder in an urban population of young adults. *Archives of General Psychiatry* 48:216–222.

Breslau, N, Kessler, RC. (2001): The stressor criterion in DSM-IV posttraumatic stress disorder: an empirical investigation. *Biological Psychiatry*; 50:699–704.

Breslau, N, Roth, T, Rosenthal, L, Andreski, P. (1996): Sleep disturbance and psychiatric disorders: A longitudinal epidemiological study of young adults. *Biological Psychiatry* 39:411–418.

Brisman, J, Siegel, M. (1984): Bulimia and alcoholism: Two sides of the same coin? *Substance Abuse Treatment* 1:113–118.

Brotman, MA, Schmajuk, M, Rich, BA, Dickstein, AE, Guyer, E, Costello, J, et al. (2006): Prevalence, clinical correlates, and longitudinal course of severe mood dysregulation in children. *Biological Psychiatry* 60:991–997.

Brown, TA, Di Nardo, PA. Lehman, CL, Campbell, LA. (2001): Reliability of DSM-IV Anxiety and Mood Disorders: Implications for the Classification of Emotional Disorders. *Journal of Abnormal Psychology* 110:49–58.

Brugha TS, McManus S, Bankart J. (2011): Epidemiology of autism spectrum disorders in adults in the community in England. *Archives of General Psychiatry* 68:459–465.

Brumberg, JJ. (1988): *Fasting Girls: the emergence of anorexia nervosa as a modern disease*. Cambridge MA: Harvard University Press.

Bryant-Waugh, R, Markham, Ll Kreipe, RE, Walsh, T. (2010): Feeding and eating disorders in childhood. *International Journal of Eating Disorders* 43, 98–111.

Burke, JD, Waldman, I, Lahey, BB. (2010): Predictive validity of childhood oppositional defiant disorder and conduct disorder: implications for the DSM-V. *Journal of Abnormal Psychology*. 119:739–751.

Buss D. (2007): *Evolutionary psychology: The new science of the mind*. New York: Allyn & Bacon.

Campbell WK, Miller JD. (2011): *Handbook of Narcissism and Narcissistic Personality Disorder*, New York: Wiley.

Cannon, TD, Cadenhead, K, Cornblatt, B, Woods, SW, Addington, J, Walker E, et al. (2008): Prediction of psychosis in youth at high clinical risk: a multisite longitudinal study in North America. *Archives of General Psychiatry* 65:28–37.

Cantor-Graae, E, Selten, JP. (2005): Schizophrenia and migration: A meta-analysis and review. *American Journal of Psychiatry* 162:12–24.

Cardno, AG, Rijsdijk, FV, Sham, PC. (2002): A twin study of genetic relationships between psychotic symptoms. *American Journal of Psychiatry* 159:539–545.

Carlat, D. (2010): *Unhinged*. New York: Free Press.

Carlson, G. (2011): Will the child with mania please stand up? *British Journal of Psychiatry*198:171–172.

Carpenter, WT. (2009): Anticipating DSM-V: Should psychosis risk become a diagnostic class? *Schizophrenia Bulletin* 35:841–843.

Carroy, J, Plas, R. (2000): How Pierre Janet used pathological psychology to save the philosophical self. *Journal of the History of the Behavioral Sciences* 36:231–240.

Chanen, AM, Jovey, M, McCutcheon, LK, Jackson, HJ, McGorry, PD. (2008): Borderline Personality Disorder in young people and the prospects for prevention and early intervention. *Current Psychiatry Reviews* 4:48–57.

Chang, K. (2007): Adult bipolar disorder is continuous with pediatric bipolar disorder. *Canadian Journal of Psychiatry* 52:418–425.

Clarkin, JF, Huprich, SK. (2011): Do DSM-V Personality Disorder Proposals meet Criteria for Clinical Utility? *Journal of Personality Disorders* 25:192–205.

Cleckley, H. (1964): *The Mask of Sanity*. 4th edition. St. Louis: Mosby.

Coccaro, E. (2010): A family history study of intermittent explosive disorder *Journal of Psychiatric Research* 44:1101–1105.

Cohen-Kettenis, PT, Owen, A, Kaijser, VG, Bradley, S J, Zucker, KJ. (2003): Demographic Characteristics, Social Competence, and Behavior Problems in Children With Gender Identity Disorder: A Cross-National, Cross-Clinic Comparative Analysis. *Journal of Abnormal Child Psychology* 31:41–53.

Coid, J, Ullrich (2010): Antisocial personality disorder is on a continuum with psychopathy. *Comprehensive Psychiatry* 51:426–433.

Coid, J, Yang, M, Tyrer, P, Roberts, A, Ullrich, S. (2006): Prevalence and correlates of personality disorder in Great Britain. *British Journal of Psychiatry* 188:423–431.

Comer JS, Mojtabai R, Olfson M. (2011): National trends in the antipsychotic treatment of psychiatric outpatients with anxiety disorders. *American Journal of Psychiatry*. 168:1057–1065.

Compton, WM, Thomas, YF, Stinson, FS, Grant, BF. (2007): Prevalence, correlates, disability, and comorbidity of DSM-IV drug abuse and dependence in the United States: Results from the National Epidemiologic Survey on Alcohol and Related Conditions. *Archives of General Psychiatry* 64:566–576.

Conners, KC, Lett, JL. (1999): *Attention-Deficit Hyperactivity Disorder in Adults and Children*. Kansas City, MO: Compact Clinicals.

Conrad, P. (2007): *The Medicalization of Society*, Baltimore, MD: John Hopkins University Press.

Cooper, JE, Kendell, RE, Gurland, BJ. (1972): *Psychiatric Diagnosis in New York and London*. London: Oxford University Press.

Copeland, WE, Shanahan, L, Costello, EJ, Angold, A. (2009): Childhood and adolescent psychiatric disorders as predictors of young adult disorders. *Archives of General Psychiatry.* 66:764–772.

Corrigan, PW, ed. (2005): *On the Stigma of Mental Illness: Practical Strategies for Research and Social Change.* Washington, DC: American Psychological Association.

Coryell, W, Solomon, D, Leon, A, Fiedorowicz, JG, Schettler, P, Judd, L, et al. (2009): Does major depressive disorder change with age? *Psychological Medicine* 39:1689–1695.

Cosgrove, L, Krimsky, S. (2012): A Comparison of DSM-IV and DSM-5 panel members' financial associations with industry: a pernicious problem persists. *PLoS Med* 9: e1001190. doi:10.1371/journal.pmed.1001190.

Costa, PT, Widiger, TA. Eds. (2001): *Personality Disorders and the Five Factor Model of Personality* (2nd ed.). Washington, DC: American Psychological Association.

Costello, EJ. (2009): Jane Costello resignation letter from DSM-V. http://www.scribd.com/doc/17162466/, accessed August 6, 2012.

Costello, EJ, Egger, H, Angold, A. (2005):10-Year Research Update Review: The Epidemiology of Child and Adolescent Psychiatric Disorders: I. Methods and Public Health Burden. *Journal of the American Academy of Child & Adolescent Psychiatry* 44:972–986.

Costello, EJ, Mustillo, S, Erkanli, A, Keeler, G, Angold, A. (2003): Prevalence and development of psychiatric disorders in childhood and adolescence. *Archives of General Psychiatry;* 60:837–844.

Craddock, N, Owen, MJ. (2005): The beginning of the end for the Kraepelinian dichotomy. *British Journal of Psychiatry* 186:364–366.

Crandall, CS. (1988): Social contagion of binge eating. *Journal of Personality and Social Psychology* 55:588–598.

Crawford, M, Koldobksy, N, Tyrer, P. (2011): Classifying personality disorder according to severity. *Journal of Personality Disorders* 25:321–330.

Cronbach, LJ, Meehl, PE. (1951): Construct validity in psychological tests. *Psychological Bulletin* 52:281–302.

Crowell, SE, Beauchaine, T, Linehan, MM. (2009): A biosocial developmental model of borderline personality: elaborating and extending Linehan's theory. *Psychological Bulletin.* 135:495–510.

Culbertson, LR. (1997): Depression and Gender: An International Review. *American Psychologist* 52:25–31.

Cumyn, L, French, L, Hechtman L. (2009): Comorbidity in adults With Attention-Deficit Hyperactivity Disorder. *Canadian Journal of Psychiatry.* 54:673–683.

Cytryn, D, Mckew D. (1996): *Growing Up Sad: Childhood Depression and Its Treatment.* New York: Norton.

Davidson, JRT, Hughes, DL, George, LK, Blazer, DG. (1993): The epidemiology of social phobia: findings from the Duke Epidemiological Catchment Area Study. *Psychological Medicine* 23:709–718.

Derogaitis, LR. (1975): *The SCL-90-R*. Baltimore, MD: Clinical Psychometric Research.

Dimsdale, JE, Xin, Y, Kleinman, A, Patel, V, Narrow, WE, Sirvatka, PJ, et al. (2009): *Somatic Presentations of Mental Disorders: Refining the Research Agenda for DSM-5*. Arlington, VA: American Psychiatric Association.

Doidge, N, Simon, B, Brauer, L, Grant, DC, First, M, Brunshaw, J, et al. (2002): Psychoanalytic patients in the U.S., Canada, and Australia: I. DSM-III-R disorders, indications, previous treatment, medications, and length of treatment. *Journal of the American Psychoanalytic Association*. 50:575–614.

Duffy, A. (2007): Does bipolar disorder exist in children? A selective review. *Canadian Journal of Psychiatry*; 52:409–417.

Duffy, A, Alda, M, Hajek, T, & Grof, P. (2009): Early course of bipolar disorder in high-risk offspring: Prospective study. *The British Journal of Psychiatry* 195:457–458.

Dunner, DI, Tay, KL. (1993): Diagnostic reliability of the history of hypomania in bipolar II patients and patients with major depression. *Comprehensive Psychiatry* 34:303–307.

During, EH. Elahi, FM. Taieb, O. Moro, M-R. Baubet, T. (2011): A critical review of dissociative trance and possession disorders: etiological diagnostic and nosological issues. *Canadian Journal of Psychiatry*. 56:235–242.

Dutta, R, Murray, RM. (2010): A life-course approach to psychosis: outcome and cultural variation. In Millon, T, Krueger, R, Simonsen, E. (Eds.). *Contemporary Directions in Psychopathology: Scientific foundations of the DSM-V and ICD-11*. New York: Guilford Press, pp. 515–522.

Eisenberg, L. (1977): Distinctions between professional and popular ideas of sickness. *Culture, Medicine and Psychiatry* 1:9–23.

Elkin, I, Shea, T, Watkins, JT, Imber, SD. (1989): National Institute of Mental Health Treatment of Depression Collaborative Research Program: general effectiveness of treatments, *Archives of General Psychiatry* 46:971–982.

Endicott, J, Spitzer, RL. (1978): A diagnostic interview: the schedule for affective disorders and schizophrenia. *Archives of General Psychiatry* 35:837–844.

Endicott, J, Spitzer, RL, Fleiss, JL, Cohen, J. (1976): The Global Assessment Scale: a procedure for measuring overall severity of psychiatric disturbance. *Archives of General Psychiatry*; 33:766–771.

Engqvist, U, Rydelius, PA. (2008): The occurrence and nature of early signs of schizophrenia and psychotic mood disorders among former child and adolescent psychiatric patients followed into adulthood. *Child and Adolescent Psychiatry and Mental Health* 2:30.

Erlenmeyer-Kirling, L, Rock, D, Roberts, SA, Janal, M, Kestenbaum, C, Cornblatt, B, et al. (2000): Attention, memory, and motor skills as childhood predictors of schizophrenia-related psychoses: The New York High-Risk Project. *American Journal of Psychiatry* 157:1416–1422.

Faedda, GL, Baldessarini, RJ, Glovinsky, IP, Austin, NB. (2004): Pediatric bipolar disorder: phenomenology and course of illness. *Bipolar Disorders.* 6:305–313.

Fairburn, C. (2011): Eating disorders, DSM–5 and clinical reality. *British Journal of Psychiatry* 198:8–9.

Faraone SV, Sergeant J, Gillberg C, Biederman J (2000): The worldwide prevalence of Attention Deficit Hyperactivity Disorder. *Journal of the American Academy of Child & Adolescent Psychiatry* 39:182–193.

Feighner, JP, Robins, E, Guze, SB, Woodruff, RA, Winokur, G, Munoz, R. (1972): Diagnostic criteria for use in psychiatric research. *Archives of General Psychiatry*; 26:57–63.

Fineberg, NA, Saxema, S, Zohar, J, Craig, KJ. (2010): Obsessive-compulsive disorder: boundary issues. In Hollander, E, Zohar, J, Sirovatka, PJ, Regier, DA. *Obsessive-Compulsive Spectrum Disorders: Refining the Research Agenda for DSM-V,* Washington DC: American Psychiatric Press, pp. 1–32.

Fink, M, Shorter, E, Taylor, ME. (2009): Catatonia Is not Schizophrenia: Kraepelin's error and the need to recognize catatonia as an independent syndrome in medical nomenclature. *Schizophrenia Bulletin* 36:314–320.

First, MB. (2005): Clinical Utility: A Prerequisite for the Adoption of a Dimensional Approach in DSM-V. *Journal of Abnormal Psychology* 114:560–564.

First, MB. (2010): Paradigm shifts and the development of the diagnostic and Statistical Manual of Mental Disorders: past experiences and future aspirations. *Canadian Journal of Psychiatry* 55:692–700.

First, MB. (2011): DSM-5 proposals for mood disorders: a cost–benefit analysis. *Current Opinion in Psychiatry* 24:1–9.

First, MB, Bell, CC, Cuthbert, B, Krystal, JH, Malison, R.Offord, DR, et al. (2002): Personality disorders and relational disorders. In Kupfer, DJ, First, MB, Regier, DA. (Eds.). *A Research Agenda for DSM-V.* Washington, DC: American Psychiatric Publishing, pp. 161–198.

First, MB, Pincus, HA, Levine, JB, Williams, JB, Ustun, B, Peele, R. (2004): Clinical utility as a criterion for revising psychiatric diagnoses. *American Journal of Psychiatry* 161:946–954.

Fombonne, E. (2009): Epidemiology of pervasive developmental disorders. *Pediatric Research*; 65:591–598.

Ford, T, Goodman, R, Meltzer, H. (2003): The British Child and Adolescent Mental Health Survey 1999: The Prevalence of DSM-IV Disorders *Journal of the American Academy of Child & Adolescent Psychiatry* 42:1203–1211.

Forman, EM, Berk, MS, Henriques, GR, Brown, GK, Beck, AT. (2004): History of multiple suicide attempts as a behavioral marker of severe psychopathology. *American Journal of Psychiatry* 161:437–443.

Frances, A. (2009a): A Warning Sign on the Road to DSM-V: Beware of Its Unintended Consequences. *Psychiatric Times* June 26.

Frances, A. (2009b): Frances Responds to APA: "Important Questions Need Answering" *Psychiatric Times* July 15.

Frances, A. (2009c): Whither DSM–V? *British Journal of Psychiatry* 195:391–392.

Frances, A. (2010a): Opening Pandora's Box: The 19 Worst Suggestions for DSM-5. *Psychiatric Times* Feb 11.

Frances, A. (2010b): How to avoid medicalizing normal grief in DSM-5. *Psychiatric Times* March 16.

Frances, A. (2010c): DSM5 and "Psychosis Risk Syndrome:" Not Ready For Prime Time. *Psychiatric Times* March 19.

Frances, A. (2010d): DSM-5 and Dimensional Diagnosis—Biting Off More Than It Can Chew. *Psychiatric Times* March 22.

Frances, A. (2010e): DSM5: "Addiction" Swallows Substance Abuse *Psychiatric Times* March 30.

Frances, A. (2010f): Psychiatric Diagnosis Gone Wild: The "Epidemic" Of Childhood Bipolar Disorder *Psychiatric Times* April 8.

Frances, A, Spitzer, RL. (2009): A message to the DSM-V workgroup. *Psychiatric Times* July 8.

Frances, AJ, Egger, HL. (1999): Whither psychiatric diagnosis. *Australian and New Zealand Journal of Psychiatry* 33:161–165.

Frank, E, Rucci, P, Cassano, GB. (2011): One way forward for the psychiatric nomenclature: the spectrum project approach. In Regier, D, Narrow, WE, Kuhl, E, Kupfer, DJ (Eds.). *The Conceptual Evolution of DSM-5.* Washington, DC: American Psychiatric Publishing, pp. 37–58.

Frazer, P, Westhuis, D, Daley, JG, Phillips, I. (2009): How clinical social workers are using the DSM-IV: A national study, *Social Work in Mental Health* 7:335–339.

Frazier, TW, Youngstrom, EA, Speer, L, Embacher, R, Law, P, Constantino, J, et al. (2012): Validation of proposed *DSM-5* criteria for Autism Spectrum Disorder. *Journal of the American Academy of Child & Adolescent Psychiatry* 51:28–40.

Freud, S. (1957): The aetiology of hysteria. In Strachey, J. (Ed. & Trans.), *The Standard Edition of the Complete Psychological Works of Sigmund Freud.* London: Hogarth Press, Vol. 3, pp. 191–224. (Original work published 1896).

Friedman, MJ, Resick, PA, Braynt, RA, Brewin, CR. (2011): Considering PTSD for DSM-5. *Depression and Anxiety* 28:750–769.

Ganguli, M, Blacker, D, Blazer, DG, Grant, I, Jeste, DV, Paulsen, JS, et al. (2011): Classification of neurocognitive disorders in DSM-5: A work in progress. *American Journal of Geriatric Psychiatry*; 19:205–210.

Garb, H. (2005): Clinical judgment and decision making. *Annual Review of Clinical Psychology*. 1:67–89.

Garfinkel, P, Lin, E, Goering, P, Spegg, C, Goldbloom, D, Kennedy, S, et al. (1996): Should amenorrhea be required for the diagnosis of anorexia nervosa? Evidence from a Canadian community sample. *British Journal of Psychiatry* 168:500–506.

Garner, DM, Garfinkel, PE. (1980): Socio-cultural factors in the development of anorexia nervosa. *Psychological Medicine*. 10:647–656.

Geller, B, Craney, JL, Bolhofner, K, Nickelsburg, MJ, Williams, M, Zimmerman, B. (2002): Two-year prospective follow-up of children with a prepubertal and early adolescent bipolar disorder phenotype. *American Journal of Psychiatry*. 159:927–933.

Geller, B, Tillman, R, Bolhofner, K, Zimerman, B. (2008): Child bipolar i disorder: second and third episodes; predictors of 8-year outcome *Archives of General Psychiatry*. 65:1125–1133.

Ghaemi, SN, Ko, JY, Goodwin, FK. (2002): "Cade's disease" and beyond: misdiagnosis, antidepressant use, and a proposed definition for bipolar spectrum disorder. *Canadian Journal of Psychiatry* 47:125–134.

Gibbons, RD, Hur, K, Brown, CH, Davis, JM, Mann, JJ. (2012): Benefits from antidepressants: synthesis of 6-week patient-level outcomes from double-blind placebo-controlled randomized trials of fluoxetine and venlafaxine. *Archives of General Psychiatry*. 69:572–579.

Gilman, SE, Breslau, J, Trinh, NH, Fava, M. (2012): Bereavement and the diagnosis of major depressive episode in the survey or alcohol and related conditions. *Journal of Clinical Psychiatry* 73:208–215.

Gold, I (2009): Reduction in psychiatry. *Canadian Journal of Psychiatry* 54:506–512.

Goldberg, D, Goodyer, I. (2005): *The Origins and Course of Common Mental Disorders*. London: Taylor and Francis.

Goldberg, D, Kendler, KS, Sirovatka, PJ, Regier DA. (2010): *Diagnostic Issues in Depression and Generalized Anxiety Disorder: Refining the Research Agenda for DSM-5*. Arlington, VA: American Psychiatric Association.

Goldstein, RB, Black, DW, Nasrallah, A, Winokur, G. (1991): The prediction of suicide. *Archives of General Psychiatry*; 48:418–422.

Gone, JP, KIrmayer, LJ. (2010): On the wisdom of considering culture and context in psychopathology. In Millon, T, Krueger, R, Simonsen, E. (Eds.). *Contemporary Directions in Psychopathology: Scientific foundations of the DSM-V and ICD-11*. New York: Guilford Press pp. 72–96.

Goodwin, FK, Jamison, K. (2007): *Manic-Depressive Illness: Bipolar Disorder and Recurrent Depression*, 2nd edition, New York: Oxford University Press.

Gottesman, I, Gould, TD. (2003): The endophenotype concept in psychiatry: etymology and strategic intentions. *American Journal of Psychiatry* 160:636–645.

Gottesman, II, Shields, J, Hanson, DR. (1982): *Schizophrenia: the epigenetic puzzle*. Cambridge, UK: Cambridge University Press.

Grant, BF, Hasin, DS, Stinson, FS, Dawson, DA, Chou, SP, Ruan, WJ (2004a). Prevalence, Correlates, and Disability of Personality Disorders in the United States: Results From the National Epidemiologic Survey on Alcohol and Related Conditions. *Journal of Clinical Psychiatry* 65:948–958.

Grant, BF, Dawson, DA, Stinson, FS, Chou, P, Dufour, MC, Pickering, RP. (2004b): The 12-Month Prevalence and Trends in DSM–IV Alcohol Abuse and Dependence: United States, 1991–1992 and 2001–2001, *Drug and Alcohol Dependence* 74:223–234.

Green, R. (1987): *The "Sissy Boy Syndrome" and the Development of Homosexuality*. New Haven: Yale University Press.

Grilo, CM, Mitchell, JE. (2010): *Treatment of Anorexia Nervosa: Clinical Handbook*. New York: Guilford.

Groopman, J. (2007): *How Doctors Think*. New York: Houghton Mifflin.

Guy, W. (1976): *Clinical Global Impression*. ECDEU Assessment Manual for Psychopharmacology, revised National Institute of Mental Health, Rockville, MD.

Hamilton, M. (1959): *The assessment of anxiety states by rating. British Journal of Medical Psychology* 32:50–55.

Gunderson, JG. (2007): Disturbed relationships as a phenotype for Borderline Personality Disorder. *American Journal of Psychiatry* 164:1637–1640.

Gunderson, JG. (2010): Revising the borderline diagnosis for DSM-V: An alternative proposal. *Journal of Personality Disorders* 24:694–708.

Gunderson, JG, Stout, RL, McGlashan, TH, Shea, MT, Morey, LC, Grilo, CM, et al. (2011): Ten-year course of borderline personality disorder: psychopathology and function from the Collaborative Longitudinal Personality Disorders Study. *Archives of General Psychiatry* 68:827–837.

Guy, W. (1976): *ECDEU Assessment for Psychopharmacology*, Revised Edition. Rockville, MD: NIMH Publication.

Hagan, F. (2008): *Introduction to Criminology: Theories, Methods, and Criminal Behavior*, Sixth Edition. Thousand Oaks, CA: Sage.

Hamilton, MA. (1960): A psychiatric rating scale for depression. *Journal of Neurology, Neurosurgery & Psychiatry* 23:56–62.

Harding, CM, Brooks, GW, Ashikaga, T, Strauss, JS, Brier, A. (1987): Vermont Longitudinal Study of persons with severe mental illness *American Journal of Psychiatry* 143:727–735.

Hare, RD. (1993): *Without Conscience: The Disturbing World of the Psychopaths Among Us*. New York: Guilford Press.

Hare, RD, Hart, SD, Harpur, TJ. (1991): Psychopathy and the *DSM-IV* Criteria for Antisocial Personality Disorder. *Journal of Abnormal Psychology* 100:391–398.

Hasin, DS, Beseler, CL. (2009): Dimensionality of lifetime alcohol abuse, dependence and binge drinking. *Drug and Alcohol Dependence* 101:53–61.

Healy, D. (2009): *Psychiatric Drugs Explained*, 5th edition, London, Elsevier.

Healy, D, Thase, M. (2003): Is academic psychiatry for sale? *British Journal of Psychiatry* 182:388–390.

Hegelstad, W, Larsen, TK, Auestad, B, McGlashan, T. (2012): Long-Term Follow-Up of the TIPS Early Detection in Psychosis Study: Effects on 10-Year Outcome. *American Journal of Psychiatry* 169:374–380.

Helzer, JE, Kraemer, HC, Krueger, RF, Wittchen, HU, Sirovatka, PJ, Regier, DA. (2008): *Dimensional Approaches in Diagnostic Classification: Refining the Research Agenda for DSM-5*. Washington, DC: American Psychiatric Association.

Hersen, E. (2003): *Comprehensive Handbook of Psychological Assessment*. New York: Wiley.

Hollander, E, Kim, S, Braun, A, Simeon, D, Zohar, J. (2009): Cross-cutting issues and future directions for the OCD spectrum. *Psychiatry Research* 170:3–6.

Hollander, E, Zohar, J, Sirovatka, PJ, Regier, DA. (2010): *Obsessive-Compulsive Behavior Spectrum Disorders: Refining the Research Agenda for DSM-5*. Arlington, VA: American Psychiatric Association.

Hopwood, CJ, Donnellan, MB, Zanarini, MC. (2010): Temperamental and acute symptoms of borderline personality disorder: associations with normal personality traits and dynamic relations over time. *Psychological Medicine.* 40:1871–1878.

Hopwood, CJ, Malone, JC, Ansell, EB, Sanislow, CA, Grilo, CM, McGlashan, TH, et al. (2011): Personality Assessment in DSM-5: Empirical support for rating severity, style, and traits. *Journal of Personality Disorders* 25:305–320.

Horwitz, AV. (2002): *Creating Mental Illness*. Chicago, University of Chicago Press.

Horwitz, AV, Wakefield, JC. (2007): *The Loss of Sadness: How psychiatry transformed normal sorrow into depressive disorder*. New York: Oxford University Press.

Horwitz, AV, Wakefield, JC. (2012): *All We Have to Fear: Psychiatry's Transformation of Natural Anxieties into Mental Disorders* New York: Oxford University Press.

Hudson, JL, Hiripi, E, Pope, HG, Kessler, RC. (2007): The prevalence and correlates of eating disorders in the National Comorbidity Survey Replication. *Biological Psychiatry* 61:348–358.

Huerta, M, Some, L, Duncan, A, Hus, V, Lord, C (2012): Application of DSM-5 Criteria for Autism Spectrum Disorder to Three Samples of Children With DSM-IV Diagnoses of Pervasive Developmental Disorders. *American Journal of Psychiatry* 169:1056–1064.

Huprich, SK, Bornstein. RF, Schmitt, TA. (2011): Self-report methodology is insufficient for improving the assessment and classification of Axis II personality disorders. *Journal of Personality Disorders* 25:557–570.

Hyman, S. (2007): Can neuroscience be integrated into the DSM-V? *Nature Reviews Neuroscience;* 8:725–732.

Hyman, S. (2010): The diagnosis of mental disorders: the problem of reification. *Annual Review of Clinical Psychology* 6:155–179.

Hyman, S. (2011): Diagnosis of mental disorders in the light of modern genetics. In Regier, D, Narrow, WE, Kuhl, E, Kupfer, DJ. (Eds.). *The Conceptual Evolution of DSM-5.* Washington, DC. American Psychiatric Publishing, pp. 3–18.

Insel, T, Quirion, R. (2002): Psychiatry as a clinical neuroscience discipline. *JAMA: the journal of the American Medical Association* 294:2221–2224.

Insel, TR. (2009): A Strategic Plan for Research on Mental Illness Translating Scientific Opportunity Into Public Health Impact. *Archives of General Psychiatry.*66:128–133.

Insel TR, Cuthbert, B, Garvey, M, Heinssen, R. Pine, DS, Quinn, K, et al. (2010): Research Domain Criteria (RDoC): Toward a new classification framework for research on mental disorders, *American Journal of Psychiatry* 167:748–751.

Ioannidis, JPA. (2005): Why most published research findings are false. *PLoS Med* 2(8): e124.

Jablensky, A, Sartorius, N, Ernberg, G, Anker, M, Korten, A. (1992): Schizophrenia: manifestations, incidence and course in different cultures. A World Health Organization ten-country study. *Psychological Medicine,* Monograph Supplement; 20:1–97.

James, I. (2006): *Asperger's Syndrome and High Achievement: Some Very Remarkable People.* London, UK: Jessica Kingsley.

Jampala, VC, Zimmerman, M, Sierles, FS, Taylor, MA. (1992): Consumer's attitudes toward DSM-III and DSM-III-R: A 1989 survey of psychiatric educators, researchers practitioners, and senior residents. *Comprehensive Psychiatry* 33:180–185.

Janis, IL. (1972): *Victims of Groupthink.* Boston: Houghton Mifflin.

John, OP, Robins, RW, Pervin, LA. (2008): *Handbook of Personality: Theory and research.* 3rd edition, New York: Guilford.

Jones, KD. (2012): A critique of the DSM-5 field trials. *Journal of Nervous and Mental Diseases.* 200:517–519.

Kafka, MP. (2010): Hypersexual Disorder: A proposed diagnosis for DSM-V *Archives of Sexual Behavior* 39:377–400.

Kagan, J. (2012): *Psychology's Ghosts.* New Haven, CT: Yale University Press.

Kahneman, D. (2011): *Thinking Fast and Slow.* New York: MacMillan.

Kanner, L. (1943): Autistic disturbances of affective contact. *Nervous Child* 2:217–250.

Keel, PK, Brown, TA, Holm-Denoma, J, Bodell, LP. (2011): Comparison of DSM-IV versus proposed DSM-5 diagnostic criteria for eating disorders. *International Journal of Eating Disorders.* 44:553–560.

Keller, MB, Klein, DN, Hirschfeld, RM, Kocsis, JH, McCullough, JP. (1995): Results of the DSM-IV mood disorders field trial. *American Journal of Psychiatry* 152:843–849.

Kelvin, L. (1889): Electrical units of measurement in popular lectures and addresses, Vol. 1, 73. Quoted in American Association for the Advancement of Science, *Science* 19:127.

Kempler, D. (1995): *Neurocognitive disorders in aging.* Berkley CA: Sage.

Kendall, T, Pilling, S, Tyrer, P, Duggan, C, Burbeck, R, Meader, N, et al. (2009): Borderline and antisocial personality disorders: summary of NICE guidance. *BMJ* 338:292–295.

Kendell, R, Jablensky, A. (2003): Distinguishing between the validity and utility of psychiatric diagnoses. *American Journal of Psychiatry* 160:4–12.

Kendell, RE. (1975): The concept of disease and its implications for psychiatry. *British Journal of Psychiatry* 127:305–315.

Kendler, KS. (2005): "A Gene for…": The Nature of Gene Action in Psychiatric Disorders. *American Journal of Psychiatry* 162:1243–1252.

Kendler, KS, McGuire, M, Gruenberg, AM, Walsh, D. (1994): An epidemiologic, clinical, and family study of simple schizophrenia in County Roscommon, Ireland. *American Journal of Psychiatry* 151:27–34.

Kendler, KS, Walsh, D. (2007): Schizophreniform disorder, delusional disorder and psychotic disorder not otherwise specified: clinical features, outcome and familial psychopathology. *Acta Psychiatrica Scandinavica* 91:370–378.

Kendler, KS, First, MD. (2010): Alternative futures for the DSM revision process: iteration versus paradigm shift. *British Journal of Psychiatry* 197:263–265.

Kendler, KS, Muñoz, RS, Murphy, G. (2010): The Development of the Feighner Criteria: A Historical Perspective *American Journal of Psychiatry* 167:134–142.

Kennedy, N, Boydell, J, Kalidindi, S, Murray, R. (2005): Gender differences in incidence and age at onset of mania and bipolar disorder over a 35-year period in Camberwell, England. *American Journal of Psychiatry* 162:257–262.

Kessler, RC, Adler, L, Barkley, R, Biederman, J, Conners, CK. (2006): The prevalence and correlates of adult ADHD in the United States: Results from the National Comorbidity Survey replication. *American Journal of Psychiatry* 163:716–723.

Kessler, RC, Chiu, WT, Demler, O, Merikangas, KR, Walters, EE. (2005a): Prevalence, severity, and comorbidity of 12-month DSM-IV disorders in the National Comorbidity Survey Replication. *Archives of General Psychiatry* 62:617–627.

Kessler, RC, Demler, O, Frank, RG, Olfson, M, Pincus, HA, Walters, EE, et al. (2005b): Prevalence and treatment of mental disorders 1990 to 2003. *New England Journal of Medicine* 352:2515–2523.

Kessler, RC, Hwang, I, LaBrie, R, Petukhova, M, Sampson, NA, Winters, KC, et al. (2008): DSM-IV pathological gambling in the National Comorbidity Survey Replication. *Psychological Medicine*; 38:1351–1360.

Kessler, RC, Gruber, M, Hettema, JM, Hwang, I, Sampson, N, Yonkers, K. (2010): Major depression and generalized anxiety disorder in the National Comorbidity Survey follow-up survey. In Goldberg, D, Kendler, KS, Sirovatka, PJ, Regier, DA. (Eds.). *Diagnostic Issues in Depression and Generalized Anxiety Disorder: Refining the Research Agenda for DSM-V.* Washington, DC: American Psychiatric Press, pp. 139–170.

Kessler, RC, Merikangas, KR, Berglund, P, Eaton, WW, Koretz, DS, Walters, EE. (2003): Mild disorders should not be eliminated from the DSM-V. *Archives of General Psychiatry* 60:1117–1122.

Kessler, RC, Sonnega, A, Bromet, E, Hughes, M, Nelson, CB. (1995): Posttraumatic Stress Disorder in the National Comorbidity Survey. *Archives of General Psychiatry.* 52:1048–1060.

Kieling, C, Kieling, RR, Rohde, LA, Frick, PJ, Moffitt, T, Nigg, JT, et al. (2010): The age at onset of attention deficit hyperactivity disorder. *American Journal of Psychiatry* 167:14–15.

Kim, Y-R, Tyrer, P. (2010): Controversies Surrounding Classification of Personality Disorder. *Psychiatric Investigation* 7:1–8.

Kim, YS, Leventhal, BL, Koh, Y-J, Fombonne, E, Laska, EE, Lim, C, et al. (2011): Prevalence of Autism Spectrum Disorders in a Total Population Sample. *American Journal of Psychiatry* 168:904–912.

Kirsch, I, Deacon, BJ, Huedo-Medina, TB, Scoboria, A, Moore, TJ. (2008): Initial severity and antidepressant benefits: a meta-analysis of data submitted to the Food and Drug Administration. *PLoS Med* 5: e45.

Klein, DF. (1987): Anxiety reconceptualized: gleaning from pharmacological dissection—early experience with imipramine and anxiety. *Modern Problems of Pharmacopsychiatry* 22:1–35.

Klein DN, Santiago NJ. (2003): Dysthymia and chronic depression: introduction, classification, risk factors, and course. Clinical Psychology.59:807–516.

Kleinman, A. (1991): *Rethinking Psychiatry: from cultural category to personal experience* New York: Free Press.

Kleinman, A. (2012): Bereavement, culture and psychiatry, *Lancet* 379:608–609.

Klerman, G. (1986): Historical perspectives on contemporary schools of psychopathology. In Millon, T, Klerman, G (Eds.). *Contemporary Psychopathology: Towards the DSM-IV.* New York: Guilford, pp. 3–28.

Knight, RA. (2010): Is a diagnostic category for paraphilic coercive disorder defensible? *Archives of Sexual Behavior* 39:419–426.

Koenigsberg, H. (2010): Affective instability: Toward an integration of neuroscience and psychological perspectives. *Journal of Personality Disorders* 24:60–82.

Kogan, MD, Blumberg, SJ, Boyle, CA, Perrin, JM. (2009): Prevalence of Parent-Reported Diagnosis of Autism Spectrum Disorder Among Children in the US, 2007. *Pediatrics* 124:2022.

Korszun, A, Moskvina, V, Brewster, S, Craddock, N, Ferrero, F, Gill, M, et al. (2004): Familiality of symptom dimensions in depression. *Archives of General Psychiatry* 61:468–474.

Kotov, R, Ruggero, CJ, Krueger, RF, Watson, D, Yuan, Q, Zimmerman, M. (2011): New dimensions in the quantitative classification of mental illness. *Archives of General Psychiatry.* 68:1003–1011.

Kraemer, HC, Kupfer, DJ, Clarke, DE, Narrow, WE, Regier, DA. (2012): DSM-5: How reliable Is reliable enough? *American Journal of Psychiatry* 169:1.

Kraemer, HC, Noda, A, O'Hara, R. (2004): Categorical versus dimensional approaches to diagnosis: methodological challenges. *Journal of Psychiatric Research* 38:17–25.

Kraepelin, E. (1921): *Manic-Depressive Insanity and Paranoia* (R.M. Barclay, Trans.). G.M. Robertson, Ed. Edinburgh: E and S Livingstone.

Krahe, B. (2007): *The Social Psychology of Aggression.* New York: Psychology Press.

Krahn, LE, Bostwick, JM, Stonnington, CM. (2008): Looking toward DSM–V: Should Factitious Disorder become a subtype of Somatoform Disorder? *Psychosomatics* 49:277–282.

Kroenke, K, Spitzer, RL, Williams, J. (2001): The PHQ-9: Validity of a brief depression severity measure. *Journal of Gen Internal Medicine* 16:606–613.

Krueger, RF. (1999): The structure of common mental disorders. *Archives of General Psychiatry.* 56:921–926.

Krueger, R, Bezdjian, S. (2009): Enhancing research and treatment of mental disorders with dimensional concepts: toward DSM-V and ICD-11 *World Psychiatry* 8:3–6.

Krueger, RF, Clark, LA, Markon, KE, Derringer, J, Skodol, AE, Livesley, WJ. (2011): Deriving an empirical structure of personality pathology for *DSM-5. Journal of Personality Disorders* 25:170–191.

Krueger, RF, Eaton, NR, South SC, Clark, LA. (2011): Empirically derived personality disorder prototype: Bridging dimensions and categories in DSM-5. In Regier, D, Narrow, WE, Kuhl, E, Kupfer, DJ (Eds.). *The Conceptual Evolution of DSM-5.* Washington, DC: American Psychiatric Publishing, pp. 97–118.

Kuhn, TA. (1970): *The Structure of Scientific Revolutions, second edition.* Chicago: University of Chicago Press.

Kupfer, DJ, First, MB, Regier, DA. (2002): *A Research Agenda for the DSM-V.* Washington, DC: American Psychiatric Association.

Kupfer, DJ, Regier, DA. (2011): Neuroscience, clinical evidence, and the future of psychiatric classification in DSM-5. *American Journal of Psychiatry* 168:172–174.

Kutchins, H, Kirk, SA. (1997): Making Us Crazy: *DSM: The Psychiatric Bible and the Creation of Mental Disorders.* New York: Simon & Schuster.

Laing, R. (1967): *The Politics of Experience,* London, Routledge & Kegan Paul.

Lake CR, Hurwitz N. (2006): Schizoaffective disorders are psychotic mood disorders; there are no schizoaffective disorders. *Psychiatry Research* 143:255–287.

Lane, C. (2007): *Shyness.* New Haven, CT: Yale University Press.

Lawrie, SM, Hall, J, McIntosh, AM, Owens, DC, Johnstone, EC. (2010): The 'continuum of psychosis': scientifically unproven and clinically impractical. *British Journal of Psychiatry* 197:423–425.

Leibenluft, E. (2011): Severe mood dysregulation, irritability, and the diagnostic boundaries of bipolar disorder in youths. *American Journal of Psychiatry* 168:129–142.

Lenzenweger, MF, Lane, M, Loranger, AW, Kessler, RC. (2007): DSM-IV Personality Disorders in the National Comorbidity Survey Replication. *Biological Psychiatry* 62:553–556.

Leonhard, K. (1979): *The Classification of Endogenous Psychoses,* 5th ed. Translated by R Berman. New York: Irvington.

Lesage, D, Boyer, R, Grunberg, F, Morisette, R, Vanier, C, Morrisette, R .(1994): Suicide and mental disorders: a case control study of young men. *American Journal of Psychiatry* 151:1063–1068.

Leucht, S, Kane, JM, Kissling, W, Hamann, J, Etschel, E, Engel, R. (2005): Clinical implications of Brief Psychiatric Rating Scale scores *British Journal of Psychiatry* 187:366–371.

Leung, AK, Lemay, JF. (2003): Attention deficit hyperactivity disorder: an update. *Advances in Therapeutics* 20:305–318.

Lewis, L, Appleby, L. (1988): Personality disorder: the patients psychiatrists dislike. *Brit J Psychiatry* 153:44–49.

Linehan, MM. (1993): *Dialectical Behavior Therapy for Borderline Personality Disorder.* New York: Guilford.

Linscott, RJ, Allardyce, J, van Os, J. (2009): Seeking Verisimilitude in a Class: A Systematic Review of Evidence That the Criterial Clinical Symptoms of Schizophrenia Are Taxonic. *Schizophrenia Bulletin* 35:1–19.

Livesley, WJ. (2010): Confusion and Incoherence in the classification of personality disorder: Commentary on the preliminary proposals for DSM-5. *Psychological Injury and Law* 3:304–313.

Livesley, WJ. (2011a): The current state of personality disorder classification. *Journal of Personality Disorders* 25:269–278.

Livesley, WJ. (2011b): An Empirically-Based Classification of Personality Disorder. *Journal of Personality Disorders* 25:397–420.

Livesley, WJ, Jang, KL, Vernon, PA. (1998): Phenotypic and genetic structure of traits delineating personality disorder. *Archives of General Psychiatry* 55:941–948.

Lloyd-Richardson, EE, Perrine, N, Dierker, L, Kelley, ML. (2007): Characteristics and functions of non-suicidal self-injury in a community sample of adolescents. *Psychological Medicine* 37:1183–1192.

Loeber, R, Burke, JD, Lahey, BB, Winters, A, Zera, M. (2000): Oppositional Defiant and Conduct Disorder: A review of the past 10 Years, Part I. *Journal of the American Academy of Child & Adolescent Psychiatry* 39:1468–1484.

Lopez-Castroman, J, Galfalvy, H, Currier, D, Stanley, B. (2012): Personality disorder assessments in acute depressive episodes: Stability at follow-up. *Journal of Nervous and Mental Diseases* 200:526–530.

Luborsky, L. (1962): Clinicians' judgments of mental health: a proposed scale. *Archives of General Psychiatry* 7:407–417.

Lux, V, Aggen, SH. Kendler, K S. (2010): The DSM-IV definition of severity of major depression: inter-relationship and validity *Psychological Medicine* 40:1691–1701.

Lux, V, Kendler, KS. (2010): Deconstructing major depression: a validation study of the DSM-IV symptomatic criteria *Psychological Medicine* 40:1679–1690.

Lynn, SJ, Lilienfeld, SO, Merckelbach, H, Giesbrecht, T, van der Kloet, D. (2012): Dissociation and dissociative disorders : challenging conventional wisdom. *Current Directions in Psychological Science.* 21:48–53.

Manners, PJ. (2009): Gender identity disorder in adolescence: a review of the literature. *Child and Adolescent Mental Health* 14:62–68.

Manuzza, S, & Klein, RG. (2000): Long-term prognosis in attention deficit/hyperactivity disorder. *Child and Adolescent Psychiatric Clinics of North America* 9:711–726.

Martin, CS, Steinley, D, Verges, A, Sher, KJ. (2011): Letter to the Editor: The proposed 2/11 symptom algorithm for DSM-5 is too lenient. *Psychological Medicine* 41:2008–2010.

Marwaha, S, Johnson, S. (2004): Schizophrenia and employment. *Social Psychiatry and Psychiatric Epidemiology* 39:337–349.

Mataix-Cols, D, Frost, RO, Pertusa, A, Clark, LA, Saxena, S, Leckman, JF, et al. (2010): Hoarding disorder: a new diagnosis for DSM-V? *Depression & Anxiety* 27:556–572.

Maughan, B, Rowe, R, Messer, J, Goodman, R, Meltzer, H. (2004): Conduct Disorder and Oppositional Defiant Disorder in a national sample: developmental epidemiology. *Journal of Child Psychology and Psychiatry* 45:609–621.

McClellan, JM, Susser, E, King, M-C. (2007): Schizophrenia: a common disease caused by multiple rare alleles. *British Journal of Psychiatry* 190:194–199.

McCrae, RR, Terracciano, A. (2005): Personality profiles of cultures: aggregate personality traits. *Journal of Personality & Social Psychology* 89:407–425.

McDonald, C. (2004): A developmental model for similarities and dissimilarities between schizophrenia and bipolar disorder. *Schizophrenia Research* 71:405–416.

McFarlane, AC. (1989): The aetiology of post-traumatic morbidity: predisposing, precipitating, and perpetuating factors. *British Journal of Psychiatry* 154:221–228.

McGlashan, TH. (1999): Duration of untreated psychosis in first-episode schizophrenia: marker or determinant of course? *Biological Psychiatry* 46:899–907.

McGlashan, TH, Zipursky, RB, Perkins, D, Addington, J. (2006): Randomized, double-blind trial of olanzapine versus placebo in patients prodromally symptomatic for psychosis. *American Journal of Psychiatry* 163:790–799.

McGee, RA, Clark, SE, Symons, DK. (2000): Does the Conners' Continuous Performance Test aid in ADHD diagnosis? *Journal of Abnormal Child Psychology* 28:415–424.

McGirr, A, Paris, J, Lesage, A, Renaud, J, Turecki G. (2007): Risk factors for suicide completion in borderline personality disorder: a case-control study of cluster B comorbidity and impulsive aggression. *Journal of Clinical Psychiatry* 68:721–729.

McGlashan, TH, Johanessen, JO. (1996): Early detection and intervention with schizophrenia: rationale. *Schizophrenia Bulletin* 22:201–222.

McGorry, PD, Nelson, B, Goldstone, S, Yung, A. (2010): Clinical staging: a heuristic and practical strategy for new research and better health and social outcomes for psychotic and related mood disorders. *Canadian Journal of Psychiatry* 55:486–497.

McGregor, E, Núñez, M, Cebula, K, Gomez, J. (2008): *Autism: An Integrated View from Neurocognitive, Clinical, Intervention Research*, Oxford: Blackwell.

McHugh, PR. (2005): *The Mind Has Mountains*, Baltimore, MD: Johns Hopkins Press.

McLaughlin, KA, Green, JG, Hwang, I, Kessler, RC. (2012): Intermittent Explosive Disorder in the National Comorbidity Survey Replication Adolescent Supplement. *Archives of General Psychiatry.* 68:90–100.

McNally, RJ. (2003): *Remembering Trauma*. Cambridge, MA: Belknap Press/Harvard University Press.

McNally, R. (2009): Can we fix PTSD? *Depression And Anxiety.* 26:597–600.

McNally, RJ. (2011): *What is Mental Illness?* Cambridge, MA: Harvard University Press.

Merikangas, KR. Akiskal, HS, Angst, J, Greenberg, PE, Hirschfeld, RM, Petukhova, M, et al. (2007): Lifetime and 12-month prevalence of bipolar spectrum disorder in the National Comorbidity Survey Replication. *Archives of General Psychiatry* 64:543–552.

Mewton, L, Slade, T, McBride, O, Grove, R, Teeson, M (2011): An evaluation of the proposed DSM-5 alcohol use disorder criteria using Australian national data. *Addiction* 72, 811–822.

Miller, JD, Campbell, K, Pilkonis, P. (2007): Narcissistic personality disorder: relations with distress and functional impairment. *Comprehensive Psychiatry*. 48:170–177.

Miller, PR, Dasher, R, Collins, P, Griffiths, F. (2001): Inpatient diagnostic assessments:1. Accuracy of structured vs. unstructured interviews. *Psychiatry Research* 105:255–264.

Moffitt, TE. (1993): "Life-course persistent" and "adolescence-limited" antisocial behavior: a developmental taxonomy. *Psychological Review* 100:674–701.

Moffitt, TE, Caspi, A, Marrington, H, Milne, B, Melchior, M, Goldberg, D, et al. (2010): Generalized anxiety disorder and depression: childhood risk factors in a birth cohort followed to 32 years. In Goldberg, D, Kendler, KS, Sirovatka, PJ, Regier, DA (Eds.). *Diagnostic Issues in Depression and Generalized Anxiety Disorder: Refining the Research Agenda for DSM-V.* Washington, DC: American Psychiatric Press, pp. 217–240.

Moffitt, TE, Caspi, A, Taylor, A, Kokaua, J. (2009): How common are common mental disorders? Evidence that lifetime prevalence rates are doubled by prospective versus retrospective ascertainment. *Psychological Medicine* 40:899–909.

Mojtabai R, Olfson, M. (2011): Proportion of antidepressants prescribed without a psychiatric diagnosis is growing. *Health Affairs*; 30:1434–1442.

Moncrieff, J. (1997): Psychiatric Imperialism—The Medicalisation of Modern Living. *Soundings*, issue 6, London: Lawrence and Wishart.

Moran, P, Coffe, C, Romaniuk, H Olsson, C, Broschmann, R, Carlie, JB, et al. (2012): The natural history of self-harm from adolescence to young adulthood: a population-based cohort study. *Lancet* 370:236–243.

Morrison, AP, French, P, Stewart, SL, Birchwood, M. (2012): Early detection and intervention evaluation for people at risk of psychosis: multisite randomised controlled trial. *BMJ* 344: e2233.

Moynihan, R, Heath, I, Henry, D. (2002): Selling sickness: the pharmaceutical industry and disease mongering *BMJ* 324:886–891.

Mullins-Sweatt, S, Widiger, T. (2009): Clinical utility and DSM–V. *Psychological Assessment* 21:302–312.

Murray, RM, Sham, P, Van Os, J, Zanelli, J, Cannon, M. (2004): A developmental model for similarities and dissimilarities between schizophrenia and bipolar disorder *Schizophrenia Research* 71:405–416.

Narrow, WE, First, MB, Sirovatka, PJ, Regier, DA. (2007): *Age and Gender Considerations in Psychiatric Diagnosis: A Research Agenda for DSM-V* Washington, DC: American Psychiatric Press.

Narrow, WE, Kuhl, EA. (2011): Clinical significance and disorder thresholds in DSM-V: the role of disability and distress. In Regier, D, Narrow, WE, Kuhl, E, Kupfer, DJ (Eds.). *The Conceptual Evolution of DSM-5*. Washington, DC: American Psychlatric Publishing, pp. 147–162.

Narrow, WE, Kuhl, EA, Regier, DA. (2009): DSM-V perspectives on disentangling disability from clinical significance. *World Psychiatry* 8:3–4.

Nasser, M, Katzman, M, Gordon, RA. (2001): *Eating Disorders and Cultures in Transition*. New York: Routledge.

Nathan, D. (2011): *Sibyl Exposed*. New York: Simon and Schuster.

National Institute for Health and Clinical Excellence (2007): *Depression: management of depression in primary and secondary care*. Accessed online, June 2009.

Newton-Howes, G, Tyrer, P, Johnson, T. (2006): Personality disorder and the outcome of depression: meta-analysis of published studies. *British Journal of Psychiatry* 188:13–20.

Norton, GR, Cox, BJ, Asmundson, GJ, Maser, JD. (1995): The growth of research on anxiety disorders during the 1980s. *Journal of Anxiety Disorders* 9:75–85.

O'Brien, C. (2011): Addiction and dependence in DSM-V. *Addiction* 106:866–867.

Office of Applied Studies. (2004): *Results from the 2003 National Survey on Drug Use and Health: National findings. DHHS Publication No. SMA 04–3964, NSDUH Series H-25*. Rockville, MD: Substance Abuse and Mental Health Services Administration.

Olfson, M, Blanco, C, Liu, L, Moreno, C, Laje, G. (2006): National trends in the outpatient treatment of children and adolescents with antipsychotic drugs. *Archives of General Psychiatry* 63:679–685.

Olfson, M, Crystal, S, Huang, C, Gerhard, T. (2010): Trends in antipsychotic drug use by very young, privately insured children. *Journal of the American Academy of Child & Adolescent Psychiatry* 49:13–23.

Osler, W. (1898): *The Principles and Practice of Medicine*. New York: Appleton.

Overall, JE, Gorham, DR. (1962): The Brief Psychiatric Rating Scale. *Psychological Reports*, 10, 790–812.

Pardini, DA, Frick, PJ, Moffitt, TE. (2010): Building an Evidence Base for DSM–5 Conceptualizations of Oppositional Defiant Disorder and Conduct Disorder. *Journal of Abnormal Psychology* 119:683–688.

Paris, J. (1996): A critical review of recovered memories in psychotherapy: trauma and therapy. *Canadian Journal of Psychiatry* 41:206–210.

Paris, J. (1997): Antisocial and borderline personality disorders: two separate diagnoses or two aspects of the same psychopathology? *Comprehensive Psychiatry* 38:237–242.

Paris, J. (1999): *Nature and Nurture in Psychiatry: A Predisposition-Stress Model* Washington, DC: American Psychiatric Press.

Paris, J. (2000): Predispositions, personality traits, and post-traumatic stress disorder. *Harvard Review of Psychiatry* 8:175–183.

Paris, J. (2003): *Personality Disorders Over Time*. Washington, DC: American Psychiatric Press.

Paris, J. (2005): *The Fall of an Icon: Psychoanalysis and Academic Psychiatry*. Toronto, Ontario, Canada: University of Toronto Press.

Paris, J. (2006): Predicting and preventing suicide: do we know enough to do either? *Harvard Review of Psychiatry* 14:233–240.

Paris, J. (2007): The nature of borderline personality disorder: Multiple symptoms, multiple dimensions, but one category. *Journal of Personality Disorders* 21:457–473.

Paris, J. (2008a): *Prescriptions for the Mind*. New York: Oxford University Press.

Paris, J. (2008b): *Treatment of Borderline Personality Disorder: A Guide to Evidence-Based Practice*. New York: Guilford Press.

Paris, J. (2008c): Clinical trials in personality disorders. *Psychiatric Clinics of North America* 31:517–526.

Paris, J. (2009): The Bipolar Spectrum: A Critical Perspective. *Harvard Review of Psychiatry* 17:206–213.

Paris, J. (2010a): *The Use and Misuse of Psychiatric Drugs: An Evidence-Based Critique*. London: John Wiley.

Paris, J. (2010b): Biopsychosocial models and psychiatric diagnosis. In Millon, T, Krueger, R, Simonsen, E (Eds.). *Contemporary Directions in Psychopathology: Scientific foundations of the DSM-V and ICD-11*. New York: Guilford Press, pp. 473–482.

Paris, J. (2010c): Estimating the prevalence of personality disorders. *Journal of Personality Disorders* 24:405–411.

Paris, J. (2012): *The Bipolar Spectrum: Diagnosis or Fad?* New York: Routledge.

Parker, G. (2005): Beyond major depression. *Psychological Medicine* 35:467–474.

Parker, G. (2011): Classifying clinical depression: an operational proposal. *Acta Psychiatrica Scandinavica* 123:314–316.

Parker, G. (2012): *Bipolar-II Disorder. Modelling, Measuring and Managing*. 2nd edition, Cambridge, UK: Cambridge University Press.

Parker, G, Fletcher, K, Hadzi-Pavlovic, D. (2011): Is context everything to the definition of clinical depression? a test of the Horwitz and Wakefield postulate, *Journal of Affective Disorders* 136:1034–1038.

Parker, G, Parker, K. (2003): Which antidepressants flick the switch? A review. *Australian and New Zealand Journal of Psychiatry* 37:464–468.

Patten, SB. (2008): Major depression prevalence is high, but the syndrome is a poor proxy for community populations' clinical needs. *Canadian Journal of Psychiatry* 53:411–419.

Patten, S, Paris, J. (2008): The Bipolar Spectrum--A Bridge Too Far? *Canadian Journal of Psychiatry* 53:762–768.

Perlis, RH, Miyahara, S, Marangell, LB, Wisniewski, SR. (2009): Long-Term implications of early onset in bipolar disorder: data from the first 1000 participants in the systematic treatment enhancement program for bipolar disorder (STEP-BD). *Biological Psychiatry* 55:875–881.

Philips, KA, First, MB, Pincus, HA. (2003): *Advancing DSM: Dilemmas in Psychiatric Diagnosis.* Washington, DC: American Psychiatric Association.

Pierre, JM. (2010): The borders of mental disorder in psychiatry and the DSM: past, present, and future. *Journal of Psychiatric Practice* 16:376–382.

Piper A, Merskey, H. (2004): The persistence of folly: critical examination of dissociative identity disorder. Part II. The defence and decline of multiple personality or dissociative identity disorder. *Canadian Journal of Psychiatry* 49:678–683.

Polanczyk, G, Caspi, A, Houts, R, Kollins, SH, Rhode, LA, Moffitt, TE (2010): *Journal of the American Academy of Child and Adolescent Psychiatry* 49:210–216.

Pope, HG, Lipinski, JR. (1978): Diagnosis in schizophrenia and manic-depressive illness: a reassessment of the specificity of 'schizophrenic' symptoms in the light of current research. *Archives of General Psychiatry.* 35:811–828.

Pratt, LA, Brody, DJ, Gu, Q. (2011): Antidepressant use in persons aged 12 and over: United States, 2005–2008. *NCHS data brief,* no 76. Hyattsville, MD: National Center for Health Statistics.

Prince, M. (1906): *The dissociation of a personality.* New York: Longmans, Green, & Co.

Prince, R, Tseng-Laroche, F. (1990): Culture-bound syndromes and international disease classification. *Culture, Medicine, and Psychiatry* 11:1–49.

Rabins, PV, Lyketsos, CG. (2011): A commentary on the proposed DSM revision regarding the classification of cognitive disorders. *American Journal of Geriatric Psychiatry* 19:201–204.

Raine, A, Lencz, T, Mednick, SA. (1995): *Schizotypal Personality* New York: Cambridge University Press.

Rajji, TK, Ismail, Z, Mulsant, BH. (2009): Age at onset and cognition in schizophrenia: meta-analysis. *The British Journal of Psychiatry* 195:286–293.

Rani, F, Murray, ML, Byrne, PJ, Wong, ICK. (2008): Epidemiologic Features of Antipsychotic Prescribing to Children and Adolescents in Primary Care in the United Kingdom. *Pediatrics* 121:1002–1009.

Rapoport, JL, Buchsbaum, MS, Zahn, TP, Weingartner, H, Ludlow, C, Mikkelsen EJ. (1978): Dextroamphetamine: cognitive and behavioral effects in normal prepubertal boys. *Science* 199:560–563.

Regier, DA, Narrow, WE. Clarke, DE, Kraemer, HC, Kuramoto, SJ, Kuhl, EA, Kupfer, DJ (2013): DSM-5 Field Trials in the United States and Canada, Part II: Test-Retest Reliability of Selected Categorical Diagnoses. *American Journal of Psychiatry* 170, 59–70.

Regier, DA, Narrow, WE, Kuhl, EA, Kupfer, DJ (2009): Conceptual development of DSM-V. *American Journal of Psychiatry* 166:645–650.

Regier, DA, Narrow, WE, Kuhl, EA, Kupfer, DJ. (2011): *The Conceptual Evolution of DSM-5*. Washington, DC: American Psychiatric Publishing.

Reich, W. (1933/1949): *Character Analysis*. New York: Orgone Institute Press.

Rettew, DC, Lynch, AD, Achenbach, TM, Dumenci, L, Ivanova, MY. (2009): Meta-analyses of agreement between diagnoses made from clinical evaluations and standardized diagnostic interviews. *International Journal of Methods in Psychiatric Research* 18:169–184.

Reynolds, C, Redline, S. (2010): The DSM-5 sleep-wake disorders: an update an invitation to the sleep community *Journal of Clinical Sleep Medicine* 6:9–1.

Rieber, RW. (2006): *The Bifurcation of the Self: The History and Theory of Dissociation and Its Disorders*. New York: Springer.

Rief, W, Mewes, R, Martin, A, Glaesmer, H, Brahler, E. (2011): Evaluating new proposals for the psychiatric classification of patients with multiple somatic symptoms. *Psychosomatic Medicine*. 73:760–768.

Roberts, AL, Dorhenwend, B, Aiello, AA. (2012): The stressor criterion for post-traumatic stress disorder—does it matter? *Journal of Clinical Psychiatry* 73:264–270.

Roberts, RE, Attkisson, C, Rosenblatt A. (1998): Prevalence of Psychopathology Among Children and Adolescents. *American Journal of Psychiatry* 155:715–725.

Robins, E, Guze, SB. (1970): Establishment of diagnostic validity in psychiatric illness: its application to schizophrenia. *American Journal of Psychiatry* 126:107–111.

Robins, L. (1966): *Deviant Children Grown Up*. Baltimore, MD: Williams and Wilkins.

Robins LN, Regier DA. (1991): *Psychiatric Disorders in America*. New York: Free Press.

Ronningstam, E. (2011): Narcissistic Personality Disorder in DSM-V—in support of retaining a significant diagnosis *Journal of Personality Disorders* 25:248–253.

Rosch, E, Lloyd, BB. (1978): *Cognition and Categorization*. Hillsdale, NJ: Laurence Erlbaum.

Rosen, GM, Lilienfeld, SO. (2008): Post-traumatic stress disorder: An empirical evaluation of core assumptions *Clinical Psychology Review* 28:837–868.

Rosenman, S, Korten, A, Medway, J, Evans, M. (2003): Dimensional vs. categorical diagnosis in psychosis. *Acta Psychiatrica Scandinavica* 107:378–384.

Rothman, DJ, McDonald, WJ, Berkowitz, CD, Chimonas, SC, DeAngelis, CD, Hale, RW, et al. (2009): Professional medical associations and their relationships with industry: a proposal for controlling conflict of interest. *JAMA*. 301:1367–1372.

Rottman, BM, Ahn, W-K, Woo-kyoung, Ph.D. Sanislow, CA, Kim, NS. (2009): Can clinicians recognize DSM-IV personality disorders from five-factor model descriptions of patient cases? *American Journal of Psychiatry* 166:427.

Rowe, R, Costello, EJ, Angold, A, Copeland, WE. Maughan, B. (2010): Developmental pathways in oppositional defiant disorder and conduct disorder. *Journal of Abnormal Psychology.* 119:726–738.

Røysamb, E, Kendler, KS, Tambs, K, Ørstavik, RE, Neale, MC, Aggen, SH, Reichborn-Kjennerud, T. (2011): The joint structure of DSM-IV Axis I and Axis II disorders. *Journal of Abnormal Psychology* 120:198–209.

Rummel-Kluge, C, Kissling, W. (2008): Psychoeducation in schizophrenia: new developments and approaches in the field. *Current Opinion in Psychiatry* 21:168–172.

Rush, AJ, Trivedi, MH, Wisniewski, SR, Stewart, JW, Nierenberg, AA, Thase, ME, et al. (2006): STAR*D Study Team: Bupropion-SR, sertraline, or venlafaxine-XR after failure of SSRIs for depression. *New England Journal of Medicine* 354:1231–1242.

Russ, E, Shedler, J, Bradley, R, Westen, D. (2008): Refining the construct of narcissistic personality disorder: diagnostic criteria and subtypes. *American Journal of Psychiatry* 165:1473–1481.

Russell, G. (1979): Bulimia nervosa: an ominous variant of anorexia nervosa *Psychological Medicine* 9:429–448.

Rutter, M. (2011): Child psychiatric diagnosis and classification: concepts, findings, challenges and potential. *Journal of Child Psychology and Psychiatry.* doi:10.1111/j.1469-7610.2011.02367.

Samuels, JF, Bienvenu, OJ, Cullen, B, Riddle, MA, Liang, KY, Eaton, WW, et al. (2008): Prevalence and correlates of hoarding behavior in a community-based sample *Behaviour Research and Therapy* 46:836–844.

Sanislow, CA, Pine, DS, Quinn, KJ, Kozak, MJ, Cuthbert, BN. (2010): Developing constructs for psychopathology research: research domain criteria. *Journal of Abnormal Psychology* 119:631–639.

Sapp, J. (2009): *The New Foundations of Evolution: On the Tree of Life.* New York: Oxford University Press.

Sartorius, N. (2011): Meta effects of classifying mental disorders. in Regier, D, Narrow, WE, Kuhl, E, Kupfer, DJ: *The Conceptual Evolution of DSM-5.* Washington, DC: American PsychIatric Publishing, pp. 59–80.

Saugstad, LF. (1989): Social Class, Marriage, and Fertility in Schizophrenia. *Schizophrenia Bulletin* 15:9–43.

Saunders, JB, Schuckit, MA, Sirovatka, PJ, Regier, DA. (2007): *Diagnostic Issues in Substance Use Disorders: Refining the Research Agenda for DSM-5.* Arlington, VA: American Psychiatric Association.

Saxena, S, Esparza, P, Regier, DA, Saraceno, B, Sartorius, N. (2012): *Public Health Aspects of Diagnosis and Classification of Mental and Behavioral Disorders.*

Refining the Research Agenda for DSM-5 and ICD-11. Arlington, VA: American Psychiatric Association and World Health Organization.

Schatzberg, AF, Scully, J, Kuppfer, DJ, Regier, DA. (2009): Setting the Record Straight: A Response to Frances' Commentary on DSM-V. *Psychiatric Times* July 1.

Schumm, BA. (2004): *Deep Down Things: The Breathtaking Beauty of Particle Physics.* Baltimore MD: John Hopkins University Press.

Schreiber, FR. (1973): *Sibyl.* Berkley, CA: Sage.

Scott, J, Paykel, E, Morriss, R, Bentall, R, Kinderman, P, Johnson, T. (2006): Cognitive–behavioural therapy for severe and recurrent bipolar disorders: randomised controlled trial. *British Journal of Psychiatry* 188:313–320.

Shedler, J, Beck, A, Fonagy, P, Gabbard, GO, Gunderson, J, Kernberg, O, et al. (2010): Personality Disorders in DSM-5. *American Journal of Psychiatry* 167:9.

Shelton, R, Fawcett, J. (2010): Antidepressant drug effects and depression severity: a patient-level meta-analysis. *JAMA.* 303:47–53.

Shields, AL, Howell, RT, Potter, JS, Weiss, RD. (2007): The Michigan Alcoholism Screening Test and its shortened form: A meta-analytic inquiry into score reliability. *Substance Use & Misuse* 42:1783–1800.

Shorter, E. (1993): *From Paralysis to Fatigue.* New York: Free Press.

Shorter, E. (1994): *From the Mind into the Body: Cultural Origins of Psychosomatic Disorders.* New York: Free Press.

Shorter, E. (1997): *A History of Psychiatry: From the era of the asylum to the age of Prozac.* New York: John Wiley & Sons.

Siever, LJ. (2007): Biologic factors in schizotypal personality disorders. *Acta Psychiatrica Scandinavica* 90:45–50.

Siever, LJ, Davis, KL. (1991): A psychobiological perspective on the personality disorders. *American Journal of Psychiatry* 148:1647–1658.

Simms, LJ, Prisciandaro, JJ, Krueger, RF, Goldberg, DP. (2012): The structure of depression, anxiety and somatic symptoms in primary care. *Psychological Medicine* 42:15–18.

Skodol, AE. (2010): Dimensionalizing existing personality disorder categories. In Millon, T, Krueger, R, Simonsen, E (Eds.). *Contemporary Directions in Psychopathology: Scientific foundations of the DSM-V and ICD-11.* New York: Guilford Press, pp. 372–373.

Skodol, AE, Bender, DS, Morey, LM, Clark, LA, Oldham, J, Alarcon, RD, et al. (2011a). Personality Disorder types proposed for DSM-5, *Journal of Personality Disorders.*

Skodol, AE, Grilo, CM, Keyes, KM, Geier, T, Grant, BF, Hasin, DS. (2011b): Relationship of personality disorders to the course of major depressive disorder in a nationally representative sample. *American Journal of Psychiatry.* 168:257–264.

Skodol, AE, Gunderson, JG, Shea, MT, McGlashan, TH, Morey, LC, Sanislow, CA (2005): The Collaborative Longitudinal Personality Disorders Study (CLPS): overview and implications. *Journal of Personality Disorders*, 19, 487–504.

Spiegel, D. (1994): *Dissociation: Culture, Mind And Body*. Washington, DC: American Psychiatric Press.

Spiegel, D, Loewenstein, RJ, Lewis-Fernandez, R, Sar, V, Simeon, D, Vermetten, E, et al. (2011): Dissociative Disorders In DSM-5. *Depression and Anxiety* 28:824–852.

Spitzer, RL. (1981): The diagnostic status of homosexuality in DSM-III: a reformulation of the issues, *American Journal of Psychiatry* 138:210–215.

Spitzer, RL. (1991): An outsider-insider's views about revising the DSMs. *Journal of Abnormal Psychology*. 100:294–296.

Spitzer, RL. (2003): Can some gay men and lesbians change their sexual orientation? *Archives of Sexual Behavior* 32:403–417.

Spitzer, RL. (2009): APA and DSM-V: Empty Promises. *Psychiatric Times*. July 2.

Spitzer, RL, Williams, JBW, Gibbon, M, First, MB. (1992): The Structured Clinical Interview for DSM-III-R (SCID), I: history, rationale, and description. *Archives of General Psychiatry* 49:624–629.

Spitzer, RL, First, MB, Wakefield, JC. (2007): Saving PTSD from itself in DSM-V. *Journal of Anxiety Disorders* 21:233–241.

Stein, DJ. (2001): Comorbidity in generalized anxiety disorder: implications and impact. *Journal of Clinical Psychiatry*. 63 (suppl):29–34.

Stein, DJ, Fineberg, N. (2007): *Obsessive Compulsive Disorder*. New York: Oxford University Press.

Steinberg, M, Hall, P. (1997): The SCID-D diagnostic interview and treatment planning in dissociative disorders. *Bulletin of the Menninger Clinic* 61:108–120.

Steiner, M, Steinberg, S Stewart, D, Carter, D, Berger, C, Reid, R, et al. (1995): Fluoxetine in the treatment of premenstrual dysphoria. *NEJM* 50:785–787.

Stern, A. (1938): Psychoanalytic investigation of and therapy in the borderline group of neuroses. *Psychoanalytic Quarterly* 7:467–489.

Stip, E, Letourneau, G. (2009): Psychotic Symptoms as a Continuum Between Normality and Pathology. *Canadian Journal of Psychiatry* 3:140.

Strauss, ME, Smith, GT. (2009): Construct Validity: Advances in Theory and Methodology. *Annual Review of Clinical Psychology* 5:1–25.

Sullivan, PF. (1995): Mortality in anorexia nervosa. *American Journal of Psychiatry* 152:1073–1074.

Sunderland, T, Jeste, DV, Baiyewu, O, Sirovatka, PJ, Regier, DA. (2007): *Diagnostic Issues in Dementia: Advancing the Research Agenda for DSM-5*. Arlington, VA: American Psychiatric Association.

Suominen, K, Isometsa, E, Ostamo, A, Lonnqvist, J. (2004): Level of suicidal intent predicts overall mortality and suicide after attempted suicide: a 12-year follow-up study. *BMC Psychiatry* 4:11.

Szasz, T. (1961): *The Myth of Mental Illness: Foundations of a theory of personal conduct.* New York: Hoeber-Harper.

Szatmari, P. (2004): *A Mind Apart: Understanding Children with Autism and Asperger Syndrome.* New York: Guilford.

Tambs, K, Czajkowsky, N, Roysamb, E, Neale, MC, Reichborn-Kjennerud, T, Aggen, SH, et al. (2009): Structure of genetic and environmental risk factors for dimensional representations of DSM-IV anxiety disorders. *British Journal of Psychiatry.* 195:301–307.

Tamminga, CA, Sirovatka, PJ, Regier, DA, van Os, J. (2009): *Deconstructing Psychosis: Refining the Research Agenda.* Arlington VA: American Psychiatric Association.

The International Schizophrenia Consortium (2009): Common polygenic variation contributes to risk of schizophrenia and bipolar disorder *Nature* 460:748–752.

Thigpen, CH, Cleckly, H. (1957): *The Three Faces of Eve.* New York: McGraw Hill.

Thombs, BD, de Jonge, P, Coyne, JC, Whooley, MA. (2008): Depression screening and patient outcomes in cardiovascular care: A systematic review. *JAMA.*300:2161–2171.

Thorup, A, Waltoft, Bl, Pedersen, CB, Mortensen, PB, Nordentoft, M (2007): Young males have a higher risk of developing schizophrenia: a Danish register study *Psychological Medicine* 37:479–484.

Tyrer, P, Mulder, R, Crawford, M (2011): Reclassifying personality disorders. *Lancet.* 377(9780):1814–1815.

Valenstein, M. (2006): Keeping Our Eyes on STAR*D. *American Journal of Psychiatry* 193:1484–1486.

Van Os, J. (2009): 'Salience syndrome' replaces 'schizophrenia' in DSM-V and ICD-11: Psychiatry's evidence-based entry into the 21st century? *Acta Psychiatrica Scandinavica* 120:363–372.

Wakefield, JC. (1992): Disorder as harmful dysfunction: A conceptual critique of DSM-III-R's definition of mental disorder. *Psychological Review* 99:232–247.

Wakefield, JC. (2007): What makes a mental disorder mental? *Philosophy, Psychiatry, and Psychology* 13:123–131.

Wakefield, JC. (2010a): Taking disorder seriously: a critique of psychiatric criteria for mental disorders from the harmful-dysfunction perspective. In Millon, T, Krueger, R, Simonsen, E. (Eds.). *Contemporary Directions in Psychopathology: Scientific foundations of the DSM-V and ICD-11.* New York: Guilford Press, pp.275–302.

Wakefield, JC. (2010b): Misdiagnosing normality: Psychiatry's failure to address the problem of false positive diagnoses of mental disorder in a changing professional environment. *Journal of Mental Health* 19:337–351.

Wakefield, JC. (2012): DSM-5: proposed changes to depressive disorders. *Current Medical Research & Opinion* 28, 335–343.

Wakefield, JC, First, MB. (2012): Validity of the bereavement exclusion to major depression: does the empirical evidence support the proposal to eliminate the exclusion in DSM-5? *World Psychiatry* 11:3–10.

Wakefield, JC, Horwitz, AV, Schmitz, MF. (2005): Are we overpathologizing the socially anxious? Social phobia from a harmful dysfunction perspective. *Canadian Journal of Psychiatry* 49:736–742.

Wakefield, JC, Pottick, KJ, Kirk, SA. (2002): Should the DSM-IV diagnostic criteria for conduct disorder consider social context? *American Journal of Psychiatry* 159:380–386.

Wakefield, JC, Schmitz, MF, Baer, JC. (2010): Does the DSM-IV clinical significance criterion for major depression reduce false positives? Evidence from the national comorbidity survey replication. *American Journal of Psychiatry* 167:298–304.

Wakefield JC, Schmitz MF, Baer JC (2011): Did narrowing the major depression bereavement exclusion from DSM-III-R- to DSM-IV increase validity? Evidence from the National Comorbidity Survey. *Journal of Nervous & Mental Disease.* 199:66–73.

Wakefield, JC, Schmitz, MF, First, MB, Horwitz, A. (2007): Extending the bereavement exclusion for major depression to other losses. *Archives of General Psychiatry.* 64:43–440.

Wamboldt, MZ, Beach, S, Kaslow, NJ, Heyman, RE, First, MB, Reiss, D. (2010): Describing relationship patterns in DSM-V: a preliminary proposal. In Millon, T, Krueger, R, Simonsen, E. (Eds.). *Contemporary Directions in Psychopathology: Scientific foundations of the DSM-V and ICD-11.* New York: Guilford Press, pp. 565–572.

Watters, E. (2010): *Crazy Like Us: The Globalization of the American Psyche.* New York: Free Press.

Weich, S, McBride, O, Hussey, D, Exeter, D, Brugha, T, McManus, S. (2011): Latent class analysis of co-morbidity in the Adult Psychiatric Morbidity Survey in England 2007: implications for DSM-5 and ICD-11. *Psychological Medicine.* 41:2201–2212.

Weiss, G, Hechtman, L. (1993): *Hyperactive Children Grown Up: ADHD in Children, Adolescents, and Adults,* 2nd edition, New York: Guilford.

Weissman, MM, Bland, RC, Canino, GJ, Faravelli, C, Greenwald, S, Hwu, HG, et al. (1996): Cross-national epidemiology of major depression and bipolar disorder. *JAMA* 31(276):293–299.

Weissman, MM, Klerman, GL. (1985): Gender and depression. *Trends in Neuroscience* 8:416–420.

Widiger, TA. (2011): The DSM-5 dimensional model of personality disorder: rationale and empirical support. *Journal of Personality Disorders* 25:222–234.

Widiger, TA, Frances, AJ, Pincus, HA. (1997): *DSM-IV SourceBook*. Vols 1–4. Washington, DC: American Psychiatric Association.

Widiger, TA, Samuel, DB. (2005): Diagnostic categories or dimensions? A question for the Diagnostic and Statistical Manual of Mental Disorders—Fifth Edition. *Journal of Abnormal Psychology* 114:494–504.

Widiger, TA, Simonsen, E, Sirovatka, PJ, Regier, DA. (2006): *Dimensional Models of Personality Disorders: Refining the Research Agenda for DSM-5*. Arlington, VA: American Psychiatric Association.

Williams, JBW, Gibbon, M, First, MB, Spitzer, RL, Davis, M, Borus, J, et al. (1992): The Structured Clinical Interview for DSM-III-R (SCID) II. Multi-site test-retest reliability. *Archives of General Psychiatry* 49:630–636.

Wilsnack, RW, Wilsnack, SC, Kristjanson, AF, Vogeltanz-Holm, ND, Gmel, G. (2009): Gender and alcohol consumption: patterns from the multinational GENACIS project. *Addiction*. 104:1487–1500.

Winchel, RM, Stanley, M. (1991): Self-injurious behavior: a review of the behavior and biology of self-mutilation. *American Journal of Psychiatry* 148:306–317.

Wing, JK. (2009): The use of the Present State Examination in general population surveys. *Acta Psychiatrica Scandinavica* 62:230–240.

Winokur, G, Cadoret, R, Baker, M, Dorzab, J. (1975): Depression spectrum disease versus pure depressive disease: some further data. *British Journal of Psychiatry* 127:75–79.

Winokur, G, Tsuang, M. (1975): Elation versus irritability in mania. *Comprehensive Psychiatry* 16:435–436.

Winokur, G. (1979): Unipolar depression: is it divisible into autonomous subtypes?. *Archives of General Psychiatry*. 36:47–52.

Wittchen, H-U, Gloster, AT, Beesdo-Baum, K, Fava, GA. (2010): Agoraphobia: a review of the diagnostic classificatory position and criteria. *Depression and Anxiety* 27:113–133.

Wonderlich, SA, Gordon, KH, Mitchell, JE, Crosby, RD, Engel, SG. (2009): The validity and clinical utility of Binge Eating Disorder. *International Journal of Eating Disorders* 42:687–705.

Woods, SW, Addington, J, Cadenhead, KS. (2009): Validity of the Prodromal Risk Syndrome for First Psychosis: Findings From the North American Prodrome Longitudinal Study. *Schizophrenia Bulletin* 35:894–908.

Worthen, J. (2007): *Robert Schumann: Life and death of a musician*, New Haven: Yale University Press.

World Health Organization. (1993): *International Classification of Diseases*, 10th edition: Mental Disorders, Geneva, WHO.

Wozniak, J. (2005): Recognizing and managing bipolar disorder in children. *Journal of Clinical Psychiatry*. 66 (Suppl) 1:18–23.

Young, A. (1997): *The Harmony of Illusions: Inventing Post-Traumatic Stress Disorder*. Princeton, NJ: Princeton University Press.

Yutzy, SH, Woofter, CR, Abbott, CC, Melhem, I, Parish, B. (2012): The increasing Frequency of Mania and Bipolar Disorder: Causes and Potential Negative Impacts. *Journal of Nervous and Mental Diseases*. 200:380–387.

Zanarini, MC. (1993): Borderline personality as an impulse spectrum disorder. In Paris J. (Ed.). *Borderline Personality Disorder: Etiology and Treatment*. Washington, DC: American Psychiatric Press, pp. 67–86.

Zanarini, MC, Gunderson, JG, Frankenburg, FR, Chauncey, DL. (1989): The Revised Diagnostic Interview for Borderlines: discriminating BPD from other Axis II disorders. *Journal of Personality Disorders* 3:10–18.

Zimmerman, M. (2011a): A critique of the proposed prototype rating system for personality disorders in DSM-5. *Journal of Personality Disorders* 25: 206–521.

Zimmerman, M. (2012a): Is there adequate empirical justification for radically revising the personality disorders section for DSM-5? *Personality Disorders: Theory, Research and Treatment* 3:444–457.

Zimmerman, M, Chelminski, I, Young, D, Dalyrymple, K, Martinez, J. (2011b): Does DSM-IV already capture the dimensional nature of personality disorders? *Journal of Clinical Psychiatry* doi:10.4088/JCP.11m06974.

Zimmerman, M, Chelminski, I, Young D, Dalyrymple, K, Martinez, J. (2012b): Impact of deleting 5 DSM-IV personality disorders on prevalence, comorbidity, and the association between personality disorder pathology and psychosocial morbidity. *Journal of Clinical Psychiatry* (online).

Zimmerman, M, Dalrymple, K, Chelminski, I, Young, D, Galione, JN. (2010): Recognition of irrationality of fear and the diagnosis of social anxiety disorders and specific phobia in adults" implications for criteria revision in DSM-5. *Depression & Anxiety*. 27:1044–1049.

Zimmerman, M, Emmert-Aronson, B, Brown, TA. (2011a): Concordance between a simpler definition of major depressive disorder and Diagnostic and Statistical Manual of Mental Disorders, Fourth Edition: an independent replication in an outpatient sample. *Comprehensive Psychiatry* 52:261–264.

Zimmerman, M, Galione, J. (2010): Psychiatrists' and nonpsychiatrist physicians' reported use of the DSM-IV Criteria for major depressive disorder. *Journal of Clinical Psychiatry*. 71:235–238.

Zimmerman, M, Mattia, J. (1999b): Differences between clinical and research practices in diagnosing borderline personality disorder. *American Journal of Psychiatry* 156:1570–1574.

Zimmerman, M, Pfohl, B, Stangl, D, Corenthal, C. (1986): Assessment of DSM-III personality disorders: The importance of interviewing an informant. *Journal of Clinical Psychiatry* 47:261–263.

Zimmerman, M, Rothschild, L, Chelminski, I. (2005): The prevalence of DSM-IV personality disorders in psychiatric outpatients. *American Journal of Psychiatry* 162:1911–1918.

Zoccolillo, M, Pickles, A, Quinton, D, Rutter, M. (1992): The outcome of childhood conduct disorder: implications for defining adult personality disorder and conduct disorder. *Psychological Medicine* 22:971–986.

Zorumski, R. (2009): Looking forward. In North, CS, Yutzy, SH. (Ed.). *Goodwin and Guze's Psychiatric Diagnosis.* New York: Oxford University Press, pp. xxv–xxxii.

Zucker, KJ. (2010): The DSM-5 criteria for gender identity disorder. *Archives of Sexual Behavior* 39:477–498.

Zucker, KJ, Bradley SJ. (1995): *Gender Identity Disorder and Psychosexual Problems in Children and Adolescents.* New York: Guilford Press.

INDEX

INDEX

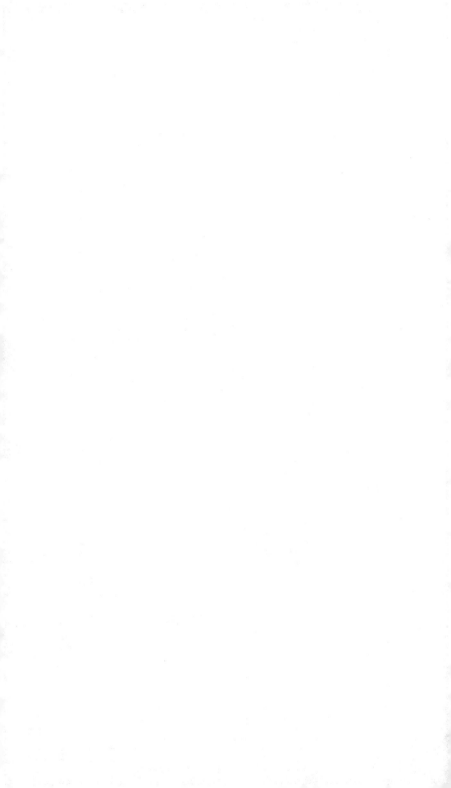